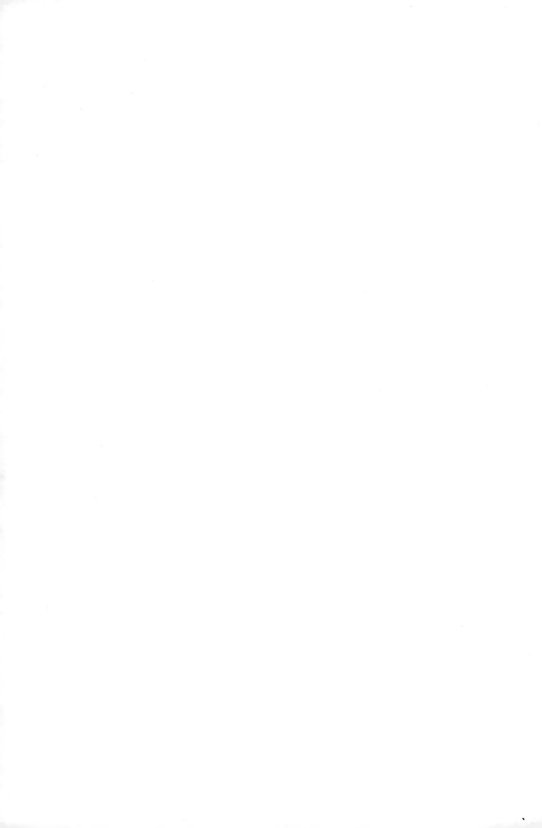

Praise for *The Change*

"An important read"

"The tag team of Milan Ross and Dr. Scott Stoll demonstrates how a new doctor and patient paradigm brought Milan a fountain of youth and Dr. Stoll fulfillment in his life's mission. *The Change* is an important read for anyone who wants to know how to transform healthcare into a more consistently successful enterprise."

–Brian Wendel
President and Founder of Forks Over Knives

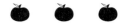

"Scientifically reliable . . . also very personal"

"Dr. Scott Stoll cares about his patients' health as sincerely as anyone I know. The story contained in these pages will show you why. Not only is the information in this book scientifically reliable, but it is also very personal. One patient documents how seven days of simply eating the right foods and listening to Dr. Stoll's message changed his life forever. This is not about hype or marketing; it's about solving health problems."

–T. Colin Campbell, PhD
Jacob Gould Schurman Professor Emeritus of
Nutritional Biochemistry, Cornell University
Coauthor of *The China Study*

"Empowering"

"Nutrient-rich food is the most powerful medicine. Thousands die needlessly each day of illnesses resulting from nutritional ignorance and food addiction. Dr. Stoll is a physician fighting to give you back control of your life and health. He doesn't just tell you to eat right; he shows you how to do it, how to make it work, and how to make it stick. *The Change* is not only a fun read but also an empowering agent of change."

–Joel Fuhrman, MD
New York Times Best-selling Author
President, Nutritional Research Foundation

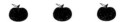

"Powerful and positive"

"*The Change* isn't just another weight-loss book. It's the true story of how Milan Ross, who once weighed over five hundred pounds, was able to take back control of his life with the help of a unique seven-day immersion program. The underlying principles of Dr. Scott Stoll's method can empower each of us to achieve lasting health and well-being. Beautifully written and utterly compelling, the anecdotes and advice offered in this book can lead to powerful and positive changes for any reader."

–John Mackey
Cofounder and Co-CEO, Whole Foods Market

"Powerful . . . .
Highly recommended"

"Dr. Scott Stoll is emerging as one of the leading voices in describing the extraordinary health benefits of lifestyle medicine in preventing and even reversing the most common chronic diseases. In this powerful book, he describes why and how. Highly recommended."

–Dean Ornish, MD
President and Founder of the
Preventive Medicine Research Institute
Clinical Professor of Medicine,
University of California, San Francisco
Author of *The Spectrum*

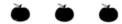

"Compelling information"

"We all need motivation and mechanisms to change. We need to be prevent-driven, not event-driven. In *The Change*, Dr. Scott Stoll brings together compelling information that can stimulate change before dangerous health events occur, while also showing us how to transform our lives after certain health conditions have taken hold. I look forward to seeing the impact this book has on its readers, and, in turn, the impact its readers have on their families, friends, and our entire culture."

–Kim Allan Williams, Sr., MD, FACC, FAHA, MASNC
President, American College of Cardiology

"Easy to read"

"The program taught by Dr. Scott Stoll and described by his patient Milan Ross in this book works for people suffering from dietary-related chronic illness, including obesity, type 2 diabetes, heart disease, intestinal issues, and inflammation. This easy to read book can lead people back to good health and youthful vigor by showing them the power of a plant-based diet of whole food."

–John McDougall, MD
Founder of the McDougall Program
National Best-selling Author

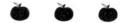

"Unique insights"

"*The Change* provides the reader with unique insights into the mindsets of teacher and student during a transformative one-week health immersion. This successful shared experience can powerfully guide anyone seeking a healthy lifestyle."

–Caldwell B. Esselstyn, Jr., MD
Author of *Prevent and Reverse Heart Disease*

MAIN SELECTION OF THE ONE SPIRIT BOOK CLUB

The Change

Milan Ross
Scott Stoll, MD

SQUAREONE
PUBLISHERS
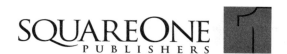

The information and advice contained in this book are based upon the research and the personal and professional experiences of the authors. They are not intended as a substitute for consulting with a healthcare professional. The publisher and authors are not responsible for any adverse effects or consequences resulting from the use of any of the suggestions or procedures discussed in this book. All matters pertaining to your physical health should be supervised by a healthcare professional. It is a sign of wisdom, not cowardice, to seek a second or third opinion.

COVER DESIGNER: Jeannie Tudor
TYPESETTER: Gary A. Rosenberg
IN-HOUSE EDITOR: Michael Weatherhead

Square One Publishers
115 Herricks Road
Garden City Park, NY 11040
(516) 535-2010 • (877) 900-BOOK
www.squareonepublishers.com

www.fullflavorvegan.com

Library of Congress Cataloging-in-Publication Data
Names: Ross, Milan, author. | Stoll, Scott, author.
Title: The change / Milan Ross and Scott Stoll, MD.
Description: Garden City Park, NY : Square One Publishers, [2016] | Includes
  bibliographical references and index.
Identifiers: LCCN 2016011005 (print) | LCCN 2016014480 (ebook) | ISBN
  9780757004322 (hbk.) | ISBN 9780757054327 (e-book)
Subjects: LCSH: Nutrition. | Weight loss. | Self-care, Health. | Food
  habits—Psychological aspects.
Classification: LCC RA784 .R675 2016 (print) | LCC RA784 (ebook) | DDC
  613.2—dc23
LC record available at https://lccn.loc.gov/2016011005

Printed in the United States of America

10   9   8   7   6   5   4   3   2   1

Contents

Acknowledgments

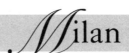

Milan

Thank you, Iris, my amazing wife, for inspiring every aspect of my life. Without your unconditional love and support, none of this would have been possible. You are my best friend, my cheerleader, and my rock. Thank you, Nigel, my wonderful son, for all the lessons you continue to teach me. I promise, we will be back at the Harry Potter ride soon, and this time I will fit in the seat. Thank you, Shalonda, Ebony, Neesa, and Georgia. I am so lucky to call you all my daughters. I love each of you more than words could ever convey.

I wrote this book in honor of my mother, Joanette Ross, and my father, James Adam Ross Sr. Mom and Dad, I miss you both so very much. Barbara, Stephanie, and Jackie, thank you for being such supportive and loving sisters. Dr. Stoll and Kristen, I am grateful beyond measure to call you my friends. I look forward to working with you both on the tasks God has placed before us. Tom Dunnam, Malissa and Chad Sarno, Lana Karpel, Allison Vernon, Wendie Pett, Kimberly

Paul, B.J. Perkins, and Nicole Jardim, thanks for being committed to helping so many people change their lives.

John Mackey, thank you for caring enough to bring the immersion program to life. Your vision continues to change the lives of countless Whole Foods Market team members. Will Paradise, I want to thank you for everything you have done for my family and me. I will never be able to repay you. Patricia Petty, thank you for allowing both me and my wife to attend an immersion retreat. Anthony Harris, thank you for always being my sounding board. I love you like a brother. I am grateful for all the love and support I have received from the entire teams at Whole Foods Highlands Ranch and Whole Foods Cherry Creek. Darcy Landis and the Whole Foods Rocky Mountain region, thank you for everything you continue to do for me. Simone Cormier and Brandon Lujan, thank you both for being amazing.

Last but certainly not least, thank you, Rudy Shur, for your insight, passion, and undeniable skill. Without your guidance, this book would not have become what it is. Michael Weatherhead, you are a rock star, my friend, plain and simple. Thanks for helping Scott and me bring our vision to life. Thanks also go out to Anthony Pomes and the rest of the Square One family. Thank you all for welcoming Scott and me with open arms, and for giving us a chance to change lives with this book.

$\mathcal{D}$r. Stoll

My precious wife, Kristen, I thank you for your eternal friendship, infinite patience, and unconditional love. We are one in all things, and life is full and rich and fun with you by my side. Thank you, my children—Dawson, Gabriel, Samuel, Joy, Elijah, and Faith—for your invaluable contributions to our family projects. Your combined support continues to encourage me to help others. Dad and Mom, thank you for your love and guidance, which always encouraged me to spend my life helping people. Linda Marino, thank you for always being my cheerleader. I am grateful to my brother, Greg, and his family, for their prayers and love. Milan and Iris, I am grateful for the work we are doing together and look forward to changing lives with you both. Heartfelt thanks go out to my friend and partner, Tom Dunnam, and his wife, Andrea. Thank you both for using your gifts to help us make it all happen.

Endless thanks go out to our amazing team: Malissa and Chad Sarno, Lana Karpel, Allison Vernon, Wendie Pett, Kimberly Paul, B.J. Perkins, Nicole Jardim, and the staff at the Naples Beach Hotel & Golf Club. We are great together. Dr. Michael Klaper and Dr. Michael Greger, thank you both for your contributions to this program, and for your friendships. Thank you, Dr. Joel Fuhrman, for your support and encouragement. Thank you, John Mackey, for your tremendous vision and backing. Thank you, Patricia Petty, for your tireless and enthusiastic assistance. Thank you, Betsy Foster, for your gracious and ongoing support. Special thanks must be extended to Steve, Jake, and David Lapp, who taught me so much about the power of unity and emotional freedom.

Finally, I would like to thank Rudy Shur, Michael Weatherhead, and the rest of the people at Square One, for their incredible talent, unwavering passion, and overall vision.

Foreword

In spite of the many amazing medical breakthroughs that have occurred over the last fifty years, our country continues to find itself in the midst of a health crisis. And while the debate over how to provide better healthcare rages on, people are dying—from heart attacks, strokes, diabetes, cancer, and so many other health conditions. The number of people directly affected by these and other serious illnesses is staggering, but these statistics tell only half the story. They don't even begin to reflect the physical, mental, and financial pain and suffering endured not only by those afflicted but also by their families. The good news is that there is something we can do to reverse what is happening to the state of our nation's health. It has nothing to do with politics, drugs, or wishful thinking. What it involves is something simple—so simple, in fact, that it is largely overlooked. It involves making the right choices when it comes to the food we eat.

Scientific research has clearly shown that a plant-based diet can reverse and, in many cases, eliminate the majority of serious, often debilitating health problems. And although this information is public knowledge, our addiction to making poor food choices continues.

The primary focus of my career as a physician has been on the connection between nutrition and good health. The well-established benefits of a highly nutritious vegan diet cannot be denied. It has been my mission to disseminate this important information to the public. Fortunately, I am not alone. In *The Change*, you will meet Dr. Scott Stoll, whose health immersion program helps guide individuals toward a healthy lifestyle through good food choices, moderate exercise, and a positive mindset. His program is attended by corporate, community, and educational groups from around the country. Businesses whose goal is to maintain healthy employees, thereby decreasing absenteeism and increasing productivity, are among his major clients.

This book offers you the opportunity to experience the seven-day "Dr. Stoll's Immersion" retreat through the eyes of Whole Foods Market employee Milan Ross. As a supporter of the program, Whole Foods sent Milan, who weighed well over four hundred pounds, on this life-changing journey. You will hear Milan's story and accompany him as he goes through his daily activities and shares his personal feelings and reactions. You will also hear Dr Stoll's story, including his inspiring lectures. You will discover how it is possible to reverse poor eating habits, even those that have been established over a lifetime, in just one week.

The Change. What an appropriate title for this book. The information it offers has provided Milan Ross and scores of others with the necessary tools to make life-altering changes. Just as important, you can apply these tools to achieve positive changes in your own life. As a physician, I can assure you that our health crisis will not go away by itself. By following the advice in this book and understanding the power of a plant-based diet, however, we can significantly reduce the number of people dealing with chronic illness. Within these pages, you will find the information to begin your own journey. The power to change is within your reach.

Wishing you the best of health,
Michael Greger, MD

The Change

$\mathcal{I}$ntroduction

At the age of thirty, my life took a truly unexpected turn. It was a life-altering experience that I would like to share with you. In this book, you will accompany me on my personal journey from skinny to obese to healthy. And when I say healthy, I am not just referring to weight. I am talking about mind, body, and soul.

It is truly extraordinary the way things happen sometimes. Who would have thought that taking a job I really didn't want with a company I didn't fully understand would be one of the best decisions of my life—second only to marrying my beautiful wife, Iris.

In October 2012, I became an employee of Whole Foods Market. It wasn't long before I found out about the great perks of working for "America's Healthiest Grocery Store." In addition to discounts on food (which can be very helpful to those who often struggle to make ends meet, as I had been struggling at the time), Whole Foods Market offered an all-expense-paid health retreat to its fulltime employees who might benefit from it. At first, the trip sounded like some type of baptism—and, in a way, it was. Unlike that religious ceremony, however, this program was focused on rediscovering yourself, determining who you would like to be, and finding a way to become that person successfully. It aimed to teach you how to eat healthfully and live healthfully.

Imagine going to a luxury resort at a tropical location for seven days to learn from the best doctors, trainers, nutritionists, and chefs, all while enjoying fun exercise on the beach every morning. That was exactly the gift Whole Foods Market gave to me. In October of 2013, one year after I'd started work, I boarded a plane and flew to Naples, Florida, to attend Dr. Stoll's Immersion program. This singular experience would change the trajectory of my entire life. Thanks to this book, you may now join me as I walk you through the same program. Step by step, I will share with you everything I did to attain my amazing results. From dealing with the emotional trauma to fighting through the withdrawal stage, you will be given an inside look at every aspect of the experience.

With the help of Dr. Scott Stoll, I will introduce you to the exact seven-day immersion process I followed. In fact, Dr. Stoll will personally take you through the ins and outs of his immersion program, detailing information that is sure to help you finally achieve the health goals you've been struggling to reach. Together we will show you how to apply this wonderful lifestyle to your everyday routine in a very practical way. From grocery shopping and cooking to exercising and staying motivated, you will be granted unprecedented access.

By sharing some of my most vulnerable and personal moments, I hope to teach others two very important facts. The first is that you are not alone. There are millions of people in this world who are all suffering from the same affliction. Obesity has grown at an alarming rate. The second is that you can change. At my heaviest, I remember feeling hopeless. I did not think I could change. Change seemed like a pipe dream. I had resolved that I, just like my mother before me and her mother before her, was destined to be obese. I had also assumed that the afflictions present throughout my family's history—afflictions such as hypertension, type 2 diabetes, and heart disease—were now my burdens as well. I couldn't have been more wrong.

As you will soon learn, the food we consume on a daily basis is a powerful force, and not only because it quite literally provides fuel for the body. It is a powerful force because of its ability to fight the progression or even onset of disease. When you eat a whole food, plant-based diet, your body receives all the nutrients it requires to operate at its optimal level. It took me over fifteen years to realize I couldn't out-train a bad diet. I had to begin eating for my health as well.

If you are reading this now and thinking that your personal struggles might be too big to overcome, or that your health is too far gone to repair, I would challenge you to allow yourself to follow *The Change* and see what happens. What I thought was going to be just another lucky on-the-job bonus—a free vacation—turned out to be a transformative event. Dr. Stoll and I now invite you to immerse yourself in the following information and become *The Change.*

GETTING ON BOARD

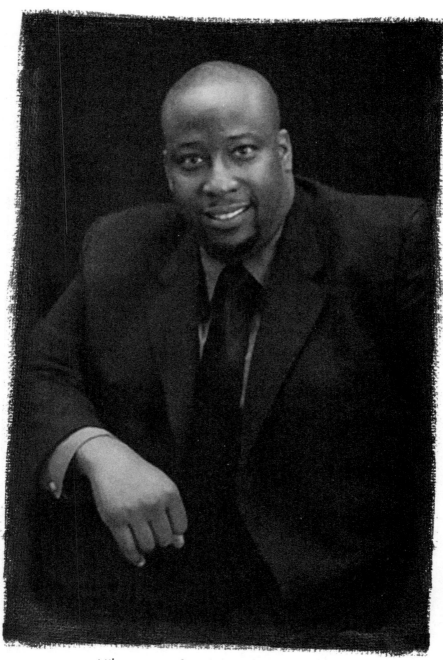

Milan as a professional, tipping the scales
at over four hundred and fifty pounds.

$\mathcal{M}$ilan's Story

My name is Milan Ross and I was once morbidly obese. I wasn't just overweight. I was so large that the everyday things most people take for granted, such as walking and standing, were huge challenges for me. At my heaviest I tipped the scales at five hundred and eighteen pounds, and the crazy thing is that I never saw the problem coming. As a child growing up in the Midwest, I was thin—very thin. Notice I didn't say I was healthy? Over the course of my journey from then to now, I have learned that being thin and being healthy are two totally different things. It wasn't too long ago that I considered them interchangeable.

Growing up in the Ross family was wonderful. We always had people over to our house for meals. My mother was a great cook, and she loved preparing food for her family and friends. She was always in the kitchen whipping up her next tasty creation, and practically every one of them would be fried or made with about a pound of butter. Just the thought of all the stuff I ate back then scares me now.

Don't get me wrong, though. My amazing mother, who was obese almost her entire adult life, did what she could with what she knew. She made sure we had a vegetable of some kind with every meal, although most of the time it would come from a can with a green giant on the front of it.

You see, like most people, my mother had picked up eating habits from her parents (my grandmother had also been obese), who had acquired them from their parents. At that time, no one was really thinking all that much about the quality of food they were eating. People just went to grocery stores and bought whatever was on the shelves—the cheaper, the better.

HOMEMADE

I grew up in Saint Louis, Missouri, the youngest of five kids, with three older sisters and one older brother. Throughout my childhood, my parents' main concern was simply putting food on the table. They didn't worry too much about how healthy that food was. If I was hungry and food was placed in front of me, I ate it. No one in my family paid attention to how much fat, sugar, or salt happened to be in our food, or thought about how large amounts of these substances might affect our bodies. As I said, my mother fried just about everything, and fried it in lard.

When it comes to discussing all the animal products my family consumed, where do I even start? Suffice it to say we ate meat, and lots of it, at every meal. I remember my mother would buy a whole hog and a whole side of beef and store them in a deep freezer in our basement. Meat wasn't a side dish at our family table. It was always the main attraction, while veggies made only small appearances on the dinner plate. We would wash it all down with a glass of red or purple Kool-Aid, which contained a full cup of sugar in every sixty-four-ounce pitcher.

The fact is that my family wasn't the only one that ate this way. Practically everyone I knew ate this way. It was the norm.

In elementary school, my fellow students and I ate mostly processed foods and drinks. The lunches served to school children back then didn't resemble a rainbow in any way. To be honest, I remember them being more gray and brown than vibrant with color. In fact, there were no salad bars to be found in any of the schools I attended as a child, including high school. There were, however, always plenty of luncheon meat, pizza, and burgers to be had—and lots of soda, chips, and candy, too. Whether at home or at school, this was the way I ate. When I became an adult, nothing changed.

As I grew into a young man, I carried with me all the eating habits I had learned as a child. I kept having lots of meat at every meal. I also continued to get pretty much all my veggies from a can. I limited fresh produce to a bag of apples or oranges. On special occasions, I would treat myself to fresh strawberries, blueberries, or peaches, but those times were rare. I knew almost nothing about how to eat in a way that would be good for my body. I simply ate what I was used to eating.

As the years passed, I became less and less active. It wasn't long before I started packing on the pounds. During my mid-twenties, I went from skinny to obese. To be honest, when I first began to gain weight, I actually thought it was pretty cool. My frame was tall and lanky. I hit a growth spurt at the age of eleven and went from five feet nine inches tall to six feet two inches tall over a summer—that's only two inches shorter than I am now. I had grown so fast that I developed scoliosis. I thought I was going to be seven feet tall and rail thin, so adding a bit of mass to my frame was a welcome change. Little did I know what lay ahead. In less than five years, I would go from being able to play sports to having to sit on the sidelines of everyday life.

REALITY CHECK

I still remember the day I recognized I was obese. This realization ingrained itself in my memory in the same way other important historical events have—like the day I married my beautiful wife, Iris, or the birth of my son, Nigel. It was December 30, 2001, my thirtieth birthday. I had invited a few friends to my house to have a few beers and celebrate with me. After a couple of drinks, we started going through some photos I had taken of us that past summer. One picture in particular hit me like a ton of bricks. It was a shot of all of us hanging out at a barbecue with no shirts on. I stood out like a sore thumb.

It wasn't that my friends were sporting six-pack abs in the photo, but I definitely looked unlike the others. I didn't appear merely out of shape. I was unrecognizable to myself. My body looked bloated and swollen. I had huge dark bags under my eyes. My skin was blotchy. I appeared tired and worn down. It was clear from the photograph that my body was reaching its breaking point. Once everyone had gone home, I pulled out the photo again and stared at it in disbelief. I was truly seeing myself for the first time.

Don't get me wrong. It wasn't that I hadn't noticed that walking or standing for any length of time had become harder for me to do, or that my body had begun to hurt in ways that should not have been familiar to a person my age. I had noticed these things, but I'd chosen to ignore them. I had other priorities. That photo, however, was a wake-up call. For whatever reason, it stopped me from continuing to pretend as though everything was okay. It removed the veil from my eyes. It caused me to stand face to face with the truth, and the truth was that I was obese—dangerously obese.

A few days later, still dwelling on the epiphany I'd had the previous night, I did an online search for the life expectancy of an African-American male born in 1971. I found that I was expected to live, under optimal conditions, to the age of about sixty-three. Given the fact that I smoked two and a half packs of cigarettes a day and weighed approximately four hundred and fifty pounds, I convinced myself I would be lucky to see the age of forty-five. Here I was, turning just thirty, thinking I had only fifteen years or so left to live—and not fifteen great years either, but rather fifteen physically and emotionally painful years.

I couldn't believe what I had done to my body. I was angry at myself because I saw my situation as completely self-inflicted. The way I had learned to eat during my childhood had produced visible effects, but I had been oblivious to them. I remembered being a child, eating just about anything I wanted to eat, never gaining a pound. I recalled every Sunday morning after church when my mom would make biscuits from scratch. I would sit at the kitchen table with a bottle of syrup and devour ten to fifteen biscuits dripping in butter and syrup, three or four eggs, and a pile of bacon. I never worried about becoming overweight. I was worrying now.

My body had changed, though I had become totally blind to this reality. But that one photograph made me see. It shocked me into recognizing the fact that I had a problem—a problem that would eventually lead me to the brink of an emotional, physical, and even spiritual breakdown.

ONE STEP FORWARD

Seeing that photograph was enough to scare me straight, at least for a while. Over the next several months, I began to buckle down. I put myself on a diet. I restricted my caloric intake and exercised daily. Granted, I was only walking on a treadmill for about twenty minutes a day, but it was working. Being more active than I had been in years, I started being able to fall asleep at a reasonable hour. My body was ready to sleep properly again. And since I no longer stayed up late, I also stopped all the late-night snacking.

Before I knew it, the pounds began to come off. I joined my local YMCA, and for the next three and a half months, I was committed. I ended up losing fifty pounds. I thought my days of being obese were soon to be a thing of the past. All my friends and family took notice of my progress.

After several months of remaining committed to my new diet plan, I decided I would allow myself a single cheat day. I told myself I would pick one day on which I would not go to the gym, and on which I would allow myself to eat anything I desired. I figured I had earned it after all the hard work I had put in. I chose the following Saturday as my cheat day. I was only at the beginning of the week, though, and still had several days to wait. I couldn't stop thinking about it. As Saturday drew closer, I felt nearly overwhelmed at the thought of a cheat day.

When Saturday finally arrived, I woke up early and started my day with breakfast at my local IHOP. I ordered what was once my "usual": the "Big Steak Omelet" with a side of bacon and an order of "Stuffed French Toast." "Yes," I said. "I would like the order of pancakes that comes with the omelet." I washed it all down with one large glass of chocolate milk and one large glass of orange juice.

After breakfast I decided to stop at the grocery store and pick up some things for the rest of my cheat day. As I made my way through the aisles, I loaded my cart with all the items I wanted. I grabbed three two-liter bottles of Pepsi, two large bags of potato chips, a half-gallon container of butter pecan ice cream, a package of Oreo cookies, and an assortment of candy bars. By the time I made it back to my car I was already mindlessly snacking on the candy bars I had grabbed at the checkout stand.

When I arrived home I promptly made my way to my favorite chair in front of the TV with one of the bags of chips I had bought in hand. I had not spent an entire Saturday in front of the television in months. I told myself that it was okay to have a day "vegging out" on the couch. After all, I had earned it. What harm could one cheat day possibly have?

After a few hours of watching the tube and polishing off the bag of chips and a liter of soda, it was time for lunch. Since I hadn't had pizza in a very long time, I decided to order pizza and wings. I called up my local Pizza Hut and placed my order: One large "Meat Lovers" pizza and sixteen honey barbecue chicken wings. When the driver arrived to drop off my food, he commented that it had been a long time since I had placed an order. He even mentioned that I looked like I had lost some weight. As I paid for my order, I told the driver that I had, in fact, been on a diet for several months, explaining to him that today was my cheat day.

After lunch, some buddies stopped by for a few beers. I hadn't drunk a beer since starting my diet. It was nice to be able to hang out with friends. Actually, it was really nice. I hadn't spent time with them in a while. I had entered a self-imposed prison of sorts, but today was a day of freedom. Now my friends and I were shooting the breeze, snacking on chips, and drinking beer. As evening turned into night and my buddies left, I settled comfortably back into my favorite chair and began to channel surf.

Somewhere around midnight I remembered the half-gallon of ice cream and package of Oreo cookies I had purchased earlier in the day. After eating the last of the pizza and wings, I turned on a movie and grabbed the ice cream and cookies. Before I knew it, it was 3 AM. As I made my way to bed I began to feel guilty for eating the way I had that day. I told myself it was only one day. One day was no big deal. I convinced myself that a cheat day is a very good thing to experience from time to time.

I awoke around noon the next day, far later than I had been getting up since starting my diet and exercise routine. I felt like I had been hit by a bus. I was exhausted. My stomach wasn't very happy with me. When I looked in the mirror I immediately noticed the swelling in my face from all the salt I had consumed the day before. Since I wasn't feeling good, I told myself I would use Sunday to recover and ended up spending all day in front of the television. This was the beginning of the end of all the hard work I had put in.

TWO STEPS BACK

Like most addicts, I found ways to rationalize whatever I wanted to do. What started out as a single cheat day turned into a cheat week, which turned into a cheat month. It wasn't long before I stopped going to the gym completely and began eating the way I had always eaten.

I went from working out every day to working out a couple of times a week to not working out at all. I was back to buying junk food and staying up late. In a month and a half, I gained back the fifty pounds I had lost plus an additional eleven pounds. I felt embarrassed and defeated. I thought about how much work it had taken me to lose fifty pounds and yet it seemed effortless to gain it all back and add more. I wanted to crawl under a rock.

The people close to me pretended not to notice that I had gained back all the weight. What surprised me most was the fact that my family and friends seemed to be relieved by my reversion to my unhealthy routine. I suppose I hadn't been much fun as a dieter. I had made myself a social outcast. I thought getting healthy meant having to isolate myself from everyone I knew. I remember one of my buddies telling me he was glad I had finally come to my senses. "If being healthy means not drinking a beer or not staying up past 9 PM, I'd rather not be healthy," he said. I remember thinking he was right.

By 2003, I had gained even more weight and was now suffering from an array of preventable chronic health conditions, including high blood pressure, high cholesterol, type 2 diabetes, diabetic neuropathy (nerve damage due to type 2 diabetes), and meralgia pares-thetica (burning thigh pain). I was taking a handful of pills every day just to function. I had pills for all my conditions, as well as pills for all the side effects those initial pills were causing. This was now my life.

In March of that year, something happened that completely freaked me out. While spending the day visiting my mother, I decided to take a nap on her couch. When I got up from my nap, my mother told me she had noticed that I would stop breathing intermittently while sleeping and then suddenly gasp for air as though I was trying not to suffocate. She said that hearing me gasp for air every couple of minutes scared her so badly that she was afraid to leave me alone. She sat there with me as I slept, making sure I was all right.

I thought breathing was something your body did automatically. Why would I stop breathing while sleeping? How long had this been going on? Could this condition kill me? I quickly performed an Inter-net search using the terms "temporarily stop breathing while sleep-ing." I discovered the problem was sleep apnea, which can contribute to heart disease and stroke. In some people, it is directly caused by obesity.

I had gained so much weight that my body was having trouble performing basic tasks such as breathing. I was terrified. I started thinking about all the other things that had been going on with my body—things I had been ignoring, like headaches and dizziness. I recalled feeling dull chest pain while getting out of the shower one day. At the time I had told myself it was probably nothing, but sud-denly I wasn't so sure. Between my weight and my two-and- a-half-pack-a-day smoking habit, I knew I wasn't doing my body any favors, and maybe this pain in my chest was its way of getting my attention again. It had been a while since I had visited the doctor. I thought it might be time to go.

I couldn't sleep the night before my doctor's appointment. I tossed and turned all night. The next morning I woke up bright and early, not because I was excited to visit the doctor's office, but because I was stressed about what my doctor might tell me about my health. I also didn't like going to the doctor because I hated the way everyone in the office would stare at me. People would gawk and whisper as though I was not standing right in front of them. As much as I didn't like going to the doctor, though, I knew I had no choice. I needed to find out the status of my health.

The appointment went about as well as I had expected it to go. For starters, I found out I was the heaviest I had ever been. I now tipped the scales at over five hundred pounds. I was also told I would more than likely need a CPAP (Continuous Positive Airway Pressure) machine (essentially a mask connected to an air pump) for my sleep apnea condition. My blood pressure was dangerously high, and my cholesterol levels were even worse than they had been at my last check-up thanks to the additional weight I'd put on.

The last thing my doctor told me was that I needed to stop smoking. She explained that the chest pain I was experiencing was my body's method of letting me know it was under too much stress. My doctor pleaded with me to improve my diet. She also strongly encouraged me to exercise daily. She offered to set me up with a specialist regarding my chest pain and sleep apnea, but I declined. I simply promised her I would eat better and exercise, and off I went.

INSIDE OUT

Over the next year I fell into a vicious circle of starve, eat, and repeat. My weight fluctuated between three hundred and fifty and four hundred and twenty-five pounds. In the summer of 2004, however, something happened that began to change me from the inside out. That was the summer I met my wife, Iris, while on a business trip to Dallas, Texas. I was working in the music industry at the time and owned a small independent record label with national distribution. In March of that year, my company, New World Records, had released the hip-hop album *From Outta Nowhere* by the rap duo D.O.A. To support the album, we had shot a music video for its first single, "Packed," and I had decided to take the group out on the road to do a promotional tour. It was during one of our tour stops in Dallas that I met Iris.

I will never forget walking into that nightclub and seeing Iris for the first time. As I sat in the V.I.P. section, I could see her hanging out with a couple of her friends, talking and laughing. I was immediately drawn to her. Something about her smile captivated me. As I gazed at her, a song came on that she really seemed to like. By chance, she happened to look up at me and smile as she started dancing. In that moment, my heart became hers to do with as she pleased.

Even though I was overweight and she was thin and fit, I decided to ask her to dance. As I signaled to her that we should hit the dance floor, she responded by nodding her head in the affirmative and making her way toward me. As she drew nearer, I immediately noticed her beautiful light green eyes. Without hesitation, she grabbed my hand. I felt like a nervous schoolboy as we made our way to the dance floor.

Within a few moments of us getting our groove on, I realized the song to which we were dancing was not the original version but rather an extended club mix. In other words, the song would not be the typical three-minute-or-so length. It could actually be a ten-minute-plus marathon of heart-pounding music. At over four hundred pounds, I quickly realized this would not end well if I could not figure out a way to get off the dance floor before I passed out. I felt as though I had already used up a week's worth of energy when all of a sudden the next song came on and Iris signaled to me that she wanted to keep dancing.

I was sweating like I'd stolen something. My back and knees were really starting to hurt. I could barely breathe, but I was determined not to let her know I was only seconds away from keeling over. By the end of the second song, all I could think about was getting off the dance floor. I quickly asked if I could buy her a drink. She graciously accepted.

We made our way back to my table and ordered drinks. As we began to talk, it was as though I had known her for years. Our conversation was effortless. Iris didn't care about my size. She connected with me in a way I had never experienced before. We spent the rest of the night laughing and chatting. Everyone else seemed to fade away. In an instant we realized we had been talking for hours.

The club was about to close for the night. As the lights came on and the mystique of the club atmosphere disappeared, I decided to take a chance. I asked Iris if she would consider having dinner with me the next day. "Yes," she said, and then she wrote her phone number down for me.

I woke up the next day like a kid on Christmas morning. I was so excited about my date with Iris that I couldn't think about anything else. Around noon, I sent her a text message asking her what time she wanted me to pick her up. I was nervous she might have changed her mind about going. Maybe the connection I had felt the night before had been a dream. A few minutes went by, and then I got a reply that said, "I am looking forward to tonight. Pick me up at 7."

The rest of the day was a blur. All I could think about was Iris. By the time evening arrived, I was excited and nervous all at once. When she opened her apartment door and I saw her, however, I instantly felt calm. She smiled and greeted me as she exited her home. We picked up exactly where we had left off the night before. There was an undeniable connection between us.

At the end of our date, we said our good-byes and promised to keep in touch. I was scheduled to leave town bright and early the next day. The next morning I woke up to a text message from Iris that simply said, "I had a great time last night. I hope you have safe travels today. Talk to you soon." Over the next six weeks Iris and I talked and texted constantly. We became best friends. I made plans to return to Texas and visit Iris when my promotional tour ended. It was during that visit that Iris and I decided to pursue a romantic relationship together. I began making plans to move to Texas. Within a few weeks of the promotional tour ending, I found commercial space and moved my record company to Dallas, Texas.

FAMILY MAN

After I moved to Dallas in 2005, Iris and I became inseparable. We got along on every level. (Even now, she still has a way of making me feel like we are the only two people in the whole world.) After a year of dating I asked her for her hand in marriage, and she granted my request. In June of 2006, we welcomed our son, Nigel, into the world. By the time Nigel was born, I had managed to lose one hundred pounds and keep the weight off. Iris and I never bought junk food or kept soda in the house. She was really into eating well and exercising regularly. She also loved to cook.

I went from eating out all the time as a single man to eating nutritious home-cooked meals as a married man. We often took long walks after dinner. Although she never asked me to lose weight, our new lifestyle was clearly having a profound effect on me, but I was still smoking two and a half packs a day. Even with the weight loss, I wasn't feeling great. Cigarettes were definitely taking their toll on me.

In the summer of 2009, while driving Nigel to preschool, something awful happened. All of a sudden I started to feel like I couldn't catch my breath. I was light-headed. I knew something was wrong. I kept getting a dull pain in my chest. After dropping Nigel off at school I called Iris and told her I was going to the emergency room. My resting heart rate was one hundred and sixty beats per minute by the time I arrived. I couldn't breathe and was on the verge of passing out. I was quickly admitted and doctors began trying to figure out what was wrong with me.

Iris got to the hospital and the attendant brought her to my room, where I was now hooked up to all sorts of monitors and being given an array of tests to determine what was going on with me. My heart rate would go from normal to an accelerated rate without warning every few minutes or so. The doctors feared my heart was being overworked, which could result in cardiac arrest. They were desperately trying to figure out the reason behind the constant jumps in my pulse.

I lay there wondering what was happening to me and tried to reassure Iris that I was going to be fine. Then my resting heart rate jumped to one hundred and seventy beats per minute and I began to black out. I could hear my wife calling for the nurse as I struggled to breathe. I could also hear all the commotion as the nurse entered the room. I was powerless to help myself. I thought I was about to lose my life.

The scariest part was the fact that the doctors couldn't explain what was causing my heart to speed up uncontrollably, even after running test after test on me. I could see the fear in Iris's eyes as they told us they didn't know what was causing the problem. I had never been so afraid.

I was released from the hospital a few days later, and as Iris and I were getting into the car she became still and began to cry. She looked at me and said, "I didn't think you were going to walk out of the hospital." I realized she had thought I might actually die. Of course, I, too, had thought I might actually die. For months after my health scare, I was afraid to be home alone with my son. I also didn't want to drive alone with him. I worried that whatever had caused the problem would return, and I didn't want to risk a recurrence that might put him in danger or distress.

For months I lived in constant fear. Although I didn't lose any significant weight after my medical crisis, I managed to quit smoking. Through the power of prayer, I have never smoked another cigarette since being released from the hospital. The weight was tougher to overcome. Over the next few years, my weight would go up and down like a yo-yo. I would lose twenty pounds and then gain thirty. I just couldn't seem to figure it all out. No matter what diet I tried, I could never maintain a healthy weight.

In March of 2011, Iris and I decided to move to Colorado. We had grown tired of all the hurricane evacuations in Texas and needed a change. Within six months of moving, Iris was diagnosed with multiple sclerosis. By early 2012, Iris began experiencing significant setbacks in regard to her overall health. We had always carried the family's insurance through her job, but now that her ability to maintain a full-time job was in question, I knew I needed to make sure we would still be covered.

Although I had moved on from being a record label owner to working as a professional voice actor, my new career didn't provide health insurance. I enjoyed recording voice-over for radio and television commercials, and it certainly paid well, but I needed to put my life in the entertainment industry on hold in order to find a job that would offer good health insurance for my whole family. Before long, I found myself an employee of Whole Foods Market.

THE TURNING POINT

In June of 2013, my wife and I decided to take Nigel to Universal Studios Orlando to celebrate his upcoming seventh birthday. Neither my wife nor my son had ever been to Florida. We planned on being in Florida on my son's actual birthday in mid-June. It was going to be awesome.

The only request my son made during our entire trip was for me to ride the Harry Potter ride with him. We had spent several weeks researching the rides prior to our vacation and Nigel had deemed the Harry Potter ride the most epic of all. He wanted to experience this epic ride with his dad. I was over four hundred and twenty pounds at the time, so in the back of my mind I worried about whether or not I would fit in one of the ride's seats. Nevertheless, I promised my son that wild horses could not stop me from getting on the Harry Potter ride with him. My health was about to make a liar of me.

On the day of our big Universal Studios Orlando visit, we arrived an hour or so before the park was scheduled to open and managed to be at the front of the line. When the gates swung open we made a bee-line for the Harry Potter ride. There was a sample of the seating on display as we approached the platform. As we made our way past the display, one of the park attendants signaled to me and asked me to step out of line. He suggested I try the seating before getting on the ride.

My son didn't know what was going on. As I went to sit down, it was obvious this wasn't going to end well. The attendant began trying to close the harness, but soon had to ask another attendant for help. I sat there for what felt like forever as these two grown men practically fractured my ribs trying to secure the harness. I realized I was not going to be able to go on this ride with my son.

After a few minutes of intense effort, the attendants stepped back and told me I would not be able to take part in the attraction. My son still didn't understand what was happening. He simply

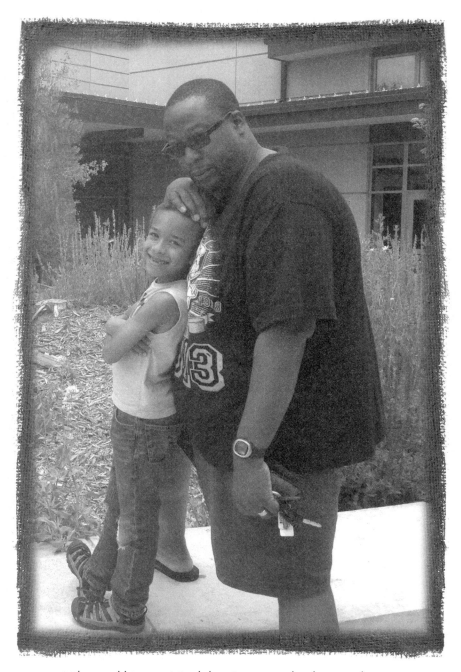

Milan and his son, Nigel, leaning on each other, as always.

heard the attendant tell me I had to leave. Nigel immediately began to cry as my wife tried to take him on the ride instead. I stood there and watched as he called out to me. I could hear him trying to explain to the man running the ride that it was his birthday, and that I had promised to go on the Harry Potter ride with him. As I stood there watching my wife practically drag my son across the platform, he screamed, "But it's my birthday! Please let my dad ride with me!"

I was devastated. Tears began to flow freely down my face, and I made myself a promise. This was going to be the last time I ever let my son down.

IMMERSION

When we returned home, I knew I had to make a permanent change, but I didn't know exactly where to begin. One day at work, Margaret—one of the assistant managers—and I were discussing health and weight loss. She mentioned an immersion health program offered by Whole Foods Market to its full-time employees who had qualifying health conditions. She explained that it was a seven-day retreat with all expenses paid, and that employees could even continue on salary that week if they used accrued vacation time. I had heard of the course, but had not given it much thought. The traumatic experience I had recently experienced with my son made me think again.

Even though I didn't fully understand what immersion meant, I asked Margaret to help me apply to the program, which had been created by a man named Scott Stoll and took place in Naples, Florida. She directed me to an internal company website, where I filled out the required paperwork and submitted my medical information for review.

Within a few weeks, I received an email from Patricia Petty, the director of the program for Whole Foods Market. The opening line of the email read, "Congratulations! You have been accepted to Dr. Stoll's Immersion program beginning October 28th." I was both excited and afraid. I immediately began to think about what this opportunity could mean to my life, to my son's life, and to my wife's life. I remember praying and thanking God for this amazing good fortune.

FEARING CHANGE

I don't think I slept for more than a few hours over the entire week preceding my trip to Florida to attend Dr. Stoll's Immersion program. I was terrified. I kept worrying about it not working, about it being one more time I failed at getting healthy. As it turned out, I already knew several people at the company who had attended this immersion course. Whole Foods Market had been facilitating this event for several years and had sent several thousand team members to it.

There were five employees at my small Denver store alone who had gone through immersion with varying results. Some of them showed no noticeable changes, while others had experienced different degrees of success. I figured at best I had a fifty-fifty chance of it working, and I was fine with those odds.

I then began to think, *What if it works? What if this is the answer I have been looking for? What will my life be like as a healthy person?* I saw myself playing basketball with my son. I saw myself going on hikes with my wife. I saw myself getting off the sidelines and living my life. The more I thought about it, the more I felt hope, which I had not felt in years.

With hope, however, came fear—fear of not knowing what life would be like after undergoing such a big change. It might sound crazy, but the very thought of being healthy was just as scary as the idea of remaining unhealthy. At least in my present state I knew exactly what to expect. I had adapted well to being obese. I had become the funny fat guy. It was my way of coping with everything.

If I actually lost weight and regained my health, then who would I be? The idea of losing weight and getting healthy permanently was frightening. The thought of certain aspects of life becoming available to me made me a little uncomfortable, as though I would be losing my identity.

At that time there were lots of things I could not fully do because of my weight and poor health. When Nigel and I would play catch, I would have to sit on a chair in the middle of our yard because I could not stand for an extended period of time without experiencing excruciating pain in my thighs. If my son threw the ball to me and I missed it, he would have to go and pick it up. This was our only way of engaging in an activity that most fathers enjoy with their sons on a regular basis. This had become our normal, and unfortunately I had accepted it. The thought of being able to take my son to the park and play catch actually scared me.

As I watched the immersion start date draw near, I was almost consumed by fear. I kept telling myself I had to do it for Nigel. I didn't want him thinking the way I was living was okay. I wanted my son to know what it was like to play catch with his dad the way other kids did with theirs. I wanted him to know what it was like to have a father who could do the things he was interested in doing, like playing basketball and football. Mostly I just wanted to be there for my son. I wanted to see him grow up and become a man. I didn't want to end up dying at a young age and miss it.

I also wanted to do it for my wife. When Iris and I met, I weighed well over four hundred pounds. I was also a very heavy smoker. I was a health crisis waiting to happen. Iris fell in love with me in spite of what I was doing to myself. I wanted her to experience a normal life with her husband. There were a lot of things we just could not do. We couldn't go for long walks together or go dancing. Iris really liked dancing, but she gave it up shortly after we got married because I simply could not do it without running out of energy almost immediately. I wanted to be able to give my wife the gift of being able to dance with her husband.

Finally, I wanted to do it for myself. After spending more than fifteen years battling obesity, I wanted off this roller coaster ride. Yes, I was terrified of the change I was about to make, but I knew I couldn't keep doing what I had been doing and survive much longer. With that, I chose to move forward. This choice didn't mean I had everything figured out. It just meant I was unwilling to remain stuck in my pattern of starve, eat, and repeat.

I drastically needed to try something different. I knew going on another diet was not going to help me over the long term. I was starting to realize that I would need to change my lifestyle if I wanted to change my life. On Monday, October 28th, I would board a plane and fly to Naples, Florida to attend Dr. Stoll's Immersion program.

Dr. Stoll's Story

As I squeezed the sixth suitcase into the last available spot in the SUV, I called for my family to hop in the car so we could head to the airport and board a plane to our seventh health immersion retreat. It was very early in the morning, and after a rather late night of packing, it was no surprise that sleep soon overtook my wife and children, giving me a quiet hour and a half in which to let my mind wander.

Of course, I thought of sunny Naples, Florida, and wondered about the people who would be there to attend the program—the life stories they would share and how they would be impacted by the week. Then I reflected back to the beginning of my own journey, when I had first thought there must be an effective way to help my patients change their lives for the better. My subsequent research into finding that elusive way would change my personal life, my family, and my practice forever. I clearly remembered the patient who had put me on a new path, startling me with her cry for help more than a decade prior.

"Doctor Stoll, please help me! I'm falling apart!" she said. These words, spoken with a nervous laugh and a half smile, underscored her true emotions, as did the hopeless look in her eye. I stopped her and asked her what exactly she had meant by "falling apart." Expecting to hear first about her back pain, and then her bad knees, and then her high blood pressure and type 2 diabetes, I was taken back when, with tears in her eyes, she began by saying, "My marriage is falling apart because the strain of my poor health has put incredible pressure on my husband. I haven't been able to see my grandchildren in three years because the travel is too hard on my body. I haven't been able to attend church in years, we are on the edge of bankruptcy because of the cost of my medications, I don't have a social life, and many of my friends rarely call anymore."

She had been looking at the floor, but now her eyes turned to me as she asked me a question that left me speechless and feeling very exposed and powerless. "What can you do to help me put my life back together again?" she said. All my years of study and training in medicine had not prepared me to answer her. I was confident and fully equipped to write a prescription, order a test, or perform a procedure, but I had no idea where to begin offering guidance to the woman sitting on the exam table.

After a long and uncomfortable silence, while my mind desperately grasped for some kind of hopeful answer, all I could come up with was an awkward promise that I would try to help her. I am sure my lack of confidence was apparent. I left the room quite shaken by the experience and plagued by my inability to offer a real solution. I asked myself what I would do for the next patient that asked me that question. Thus began a several-year research project to find out how to help people overcome or even avoid common degenerative diseases.

I began by reading most of the popular diet books on the market, from *Dr. Atkins' New Diet Revolution* to *The Zone Diet*, thinking that someone must have the answer to the problem of "falling apart." The books had compelling information and research to support their positions, but something was missing. They did not appear to have any comprehensive solution to the collateral damage of lifestyle diseases or to the diseases themselves.

In many cases, the primary goal of the diet book was weight loss, and I learned from research that the best-case scenario for long-term

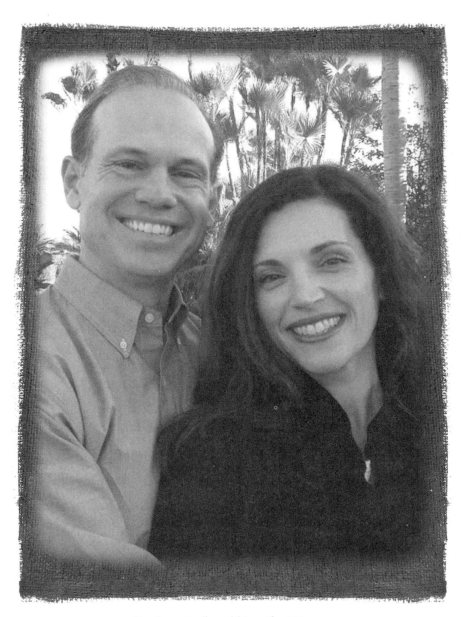

Dr. Scott Stoll and his wife, Kristen,
ready for another immersion week.

weight management from any diet was 15 percent at five years.[1] Now, how could I expect anyone to undertake a challenging project that would require sacrifice, discomfort, focus, and personal investment but had only a modest upside and an average success rate of 15 percent? I couldn't. Yet every year, approximately fifty million people begin new diets, hoping for new, easier, and different outcomes than those of the diets they followed the year before.

The fact is that yo-yo dieting leaves people heavier, sicker, hopeless, and frequently feeling shame, guilt, self-judgment, and self-condemnation. Essentially, the only thing that really gets lighter for a dieter over the years is his or her wallet.

I knew I could not recommend a diet book as the solution for my patients, so I turned my attention back to academic research as I searched for an answer. Over the course of two years, I reviewed thousands of studies and found one common thread. The body of research consistently showed that the higher the intake of plant-based food, such as vegetables, fruits, beans, etc., the healthier the body, and the more disease-resistant the body remains over time.

I visited Dr. Joel Fuhrman at his office in New Jersey. A physician who had been using nutrition to treat his patients, he showed me case after case of patients overcoming diseases I'd thought were irreversible, and these patients were actually getting healthier with age! I decided to follow this approach to illness at home with my family first. After speaking with my wife about what I had learned, she agreed to change the way she had been cooking. She had always believed her meals to be healthful, but now she knew she would have to search for a whole new set of recipes. My wife and I soon saw improvements in ourselves. We also noticed our children rarely got sick anymore—no more ear infections, no more antibiotics, and only a very rare passing cold.

I began to use my prescription pad at my medical practice to write recipes for smoothies, lunches, and dinners. I started to see amazing results in some of my patients, including the reversal of high blood pressure and type 2 diabetes, as well as the discontinuation of many medications. For the first time, many of my patients reported resolution of pain and significant long-term weight loss without feelings of deprivation or sacrifice. One patient even lost over one hundred pounds without exercising and reported that she no longer felt hungry all the time. She had literally eaten her way to a healthy weight.

In light of all this success, my wife and I decided to host our first one-day health program. We held it in a rented conference room at DeSales University, located in Center Valley, Pennsylvania, close to our home. We promoted the seminar at my hospital, local churches, and bookstores, and told our friends and family about it. Nearly two hundred people ended up attending. It featured lectures on the science of health, an exercise session, a culinary class given by my wife, and a delicious plant-based lunch. Essentially, attendants immersed themselves in a new lifestyle over the course of an entire day. This idea of immersion was a seed planted in fertile soil.

A BRIEF HISTORY OF HEALTH IMMERSION

As I continued driving to the airport, recalling the origins of the program I was about to lead yet again, I began thinking about the history of health immersion itself. The concept of health immersion was not new or untested when my wife and I ran our first retreat— far from it.

In 1975, Nathan Pritikin, an inventor in the fields of physics, chemistry, and electronics, opened the first four-week health immersion program. His visionary immersion program was, in fact, born out of his own personal battle with disease. At the age of forty-one, Nathan was diagnosed with severe heart disease and refused to accept the bleak prognosis of a short life. He analyzed all the research he could find, looking for a solution, and discovered that heart disease could be treated effectively with lifestyle changes. In light of this finding, he decided to immerse himself in a new way of being.

He removed processed food from his diet and shifted to plant-based nutrition with occasional animal products, while also incorporating exercise and stress management into his daily routine. In doing so, he lowered his cholesterol significantly, reversed his heart disease, and normalized his heart rate. His experience motivated him to help others. He once said in an interview, "All I am trying to do is wipe out heart disease, diabetes, and obesity." And so immersion therapy was born.

Today more than one hundred published studies have been based on his ideas, which demonstrate the fact that numerous diseases can be reversed through diet and lifestyle intervention. For example, one study showed 74 percent of type 2 diabetic patients were able to discontinue all their medications by immersing themselves in a healthy lifestyle and following a plant-based diet for just four weeks, and 44 percent of those on insulin came off insulin in the same time period.[2]

One study analyzed 1,615 participants who had been placed on a low-fat vegan diet and found that blood pressure, total cholesterol, blood sugar, and cardiovascular risk had improved significantly in just one week. Of the participants on medication for high blood pressure or elevated blood sugar (type 2 diabetes), 86.5 percent of those on high blood pressure drugs and 90.7 percent of those on diabetic drugs had seen their dosages reduced or discontinued by the end of the seven-day treatment.[3]

The concept of health immersion blossomed under the cofounder and co-CEO of Whole Foods Market, John Mackey. He was instrumental in developing a one-week immersion program to help improve the health of Whole Foods team members who were facing chronic health conditions such as heart disease, type 2 diabetes, or high blood pressure. I had been serving on the Whole Foods Scientific and Medical advisory board when I was asked to host a week-long health immersion program for Whole Foods. Of course, the idea made perfect sense to me.

The one-week program we run is a unique opportunity for people to step back from their busy schedules, bad habits, tempting food environments, and the stressors and pressures of life and recapture perspective, vision, inspiration, and motivation. Ultimately, it teaches attendees how good it feels to take care of their bodies through dietary and lifestyle changes. It is a comprehensive health education program that embraces the most up-to-date science of nutrition, achievable kinds of exercise (or, as we like to say, movement), and culinary education, encouragement, and coaching.

Food is the centerpiece of the retreat, so we work closely with the chef and kitchen staff of the hotel at which the retreat is held. Under our guidance, they prepare delicious, healthy meals for the program's participants every day. Each dish is meant to please the palate and fulfill the needs of the body. It is always a fun and uniquely transformational week, as evidenced by the incredible stories of people who altered the trajectory of their lives by attending the program, people who fundamentally changed their futures after just one week.

Symptoms of many health conditions—including type 2 diabetes, high blood pressure, rheumatoid arthritis, fibromyalgia, psoriasis, headaches, heart disease, sleep apnea, arthritic pain, chronic constipation, irritable bowel disease, and reflux, to name but a few—have frequently been eliminated by the application of the principles taught during this one week. I have personally seen much more than just minor improvement in participants' weight, blood pressure readings, and cholesterol numbers.

So many of those who have taken part in this seven-day retreat have attained healthy lives and found freedom. They have found freedom from fatigue, pain, sleep disruption, constipation, memory impairment, and decreased mobility. They have found freedom from the emotional pain associated with disease, including depression, anxiety, irritability, fear, and hopelessness. They have found freedom from the financial depletion that often accompanies disease. They have found freedom from the relationship problems associated with dealing with disease. They have found freedom from the occupational disruption caused by disease. They have found freedom from the spiritual distraction of disease. Every year, we at the immersion program hear from people whose lives have been beautifully transformed.

LUCKY NUMBER SEVEN

My mind was brought back to the present moment by a knock on the driver-side window of my car. A parking attendant was motioning his desire to hand me my parking stub. I followed his directions and pulled the car into a spot designated for extended-stay vehicles. My wife and children woke from their respective slumbers at the squeak of the brakes. Like a well-trained troop, we unloaded the bags from the car and transferred them to the airport shuttle van. We would soon be taking flight to our seventh immersion retreat.

DAY ONE

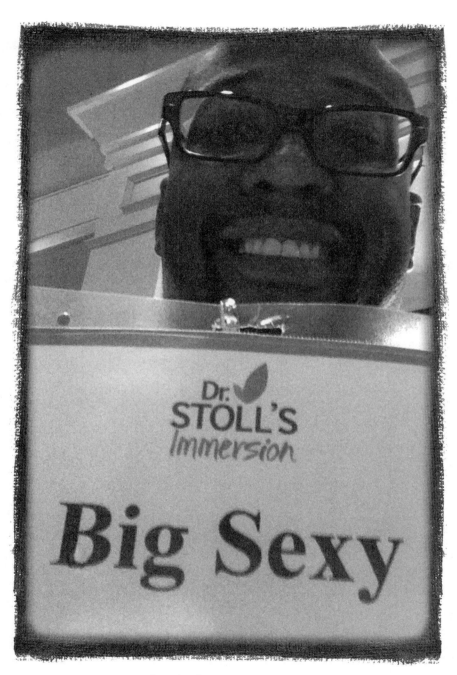

Milan checking in to immersion.

Milan's Story

I awoke in a panic on my first day of the immersion program, which would officially start upon my arrival at the hotel in Florida later that afternoon. I had hoped to get a good night's sleep prior to heading to the airport and setting off on my journey, but all I had done was toss and turn. So many questions continued to pop into my head: *Would this retreat be some sort of fat camp? If not, would I be the only overweight person there? What would my roommate be like? Would we get along? What would the food be like? What if I hated everything?* It wasn't as though I could take a taxi back to my house if I ended up not enjoying the experience. I would be stuck there for one week. Despite my obsessive thoughts, I knew I had to drag myself out of bed and get going.

My wife and son dropped me off at the airport about two hours before my flight. I think Iris could tell I was a bit nervous. As she kissed me good-bye, she whispered, "It will be okay. Just go and allow yourself to engage fully, and remember you are going to be on the beach, so have fun." I exited the car and turned to open the rear passenger-side door and kiss my son good-bye. Nigel, being a typical seven-year-old kid, asked me if I would be skinny the next time he saw me. I laughed and told him it probably wouldn't work that way. I grabbed my suitcase out of the trunk and made my way inside the airport.

I checked my bag, made it through security, and realized I still had about an hour and forty minutes before my flight was scheduled to depart. As I headed to my gate, it dawned on me: With all the excitement, I had not eaten breakfast or lunch. It was now 1 PM and I was starving. I wasn't sure what time I would be able to eat once I got to immersion, so I decided to buy something. I headed to the restaurant area to peruse the offerings.

I wish I could say I stopped at a restaurant that sold the most incredibly healthy food you've ever seen, but that wouldn't be true. Frankly, I found the only barbecue restaurant at the airport and proceeded to order a full slab of ribs with a basket of hand-cut fries. Old habits die hard. I convinced myself I was showing restraint in my decision to have water with a lemon wedge instead of a soda.

I was already feeling guilty for eating the barbecue by the time I boarded my flight about an hour later. Add to that the fact that I was now about to squeeze myself into a tiny seat on an airplane for the next several hours and you will see my immersion adventure was not starting off on particularly solid footing. I requested a lap extension belt and settled in for the flight. I could already feel the seat digging into my hips before the plane even left the ground.

At the airport in Florida, I grabbed my suitcase at baggage claim and encountered several other people who would also be attending immersion. We quickly realized we were all headed to the same place when each of us began walking toward a woman holding a sign that said "Dr. Stoll's Immersion." This woman took our names, checking her clipboard as she went along. She informed us that we would leave as soon as the remaining attendees showed up. We all stood there waiting for them, introducing ourselves to each other to pass the time. Each participant took a turn stating his or her name, Whole Foods store location, and job title. When my turn came, I said hurriedly, "Milan Ross, Highlands Ranch, front-end supervisor."

One guy, who had actually been sitting across the aisle from me on the plane, began talking to me. He asked me how long I had been with Whole Foods Market. When I told him that my one-year anniversary had just passed at the beginning of the month, he laughed and said, "You barely made the one-year-employment requirement to come to this thing!" I chuckled and told him my wife saw that fact as a sign that I was meant to attend this immersion retreat. I also mentioned that I thought the folks in charge of the program had realized how badly I needed to be there and simply made it happen. Our conversation was interrupted by the woman with the clipboard informing us that our group was ready to head to the resort.

As I checked in at the front desk of the Naples Beach Hotel & Golf Club, the clerk informed me I would be rooming with a man named Michael. Almost immediately after receiving this news, I heard a voice from behind me say, "That's me!" I turned around and was met by the friendly face and outstretched arm of my new roommate, Michael. We shook hands and officially introduced ourselves to one another. As I would soon discover, Michael was a funny, articulate guy, born and raised in a small city just across the Mississippi River from Saint Louis, Missouri, my hometown. He had a warm and outgoing personality, which made people naturally gravitate toward him.

After a few minutes of conversation, I realized Michael and I had several things in common. We were both about the same age, we both had sons, and we both struggled with health issues. He told me he had been dealing with high blood pressure and high cholesterol and was now prediabetic. As I listened to him, I thought about how similar our situations were. Although I was much larger than Michael (both taller and heavier), it was easy to understand why he and I had been paired as roommates. I was certain we would get along just fine.

Together we took notice of how beautiful the resort was. The lobby featured a relaxing beach motif and a stunning exposed-beam ceiling. The back wall had floor-to-ceiling windows. The windows not only allowed lots of natural light to flood in, but they also framed breathtaking views of the ocean, which sat about fifty yards from the back door of the hotel. It was obvious no detail had been overlooked.

After checking in, I ventured a bit farther into the hotel lobby, where I saw the "Dr. Stoll's Immersion" registration table. The registration staff was cheerful and fun. As I approached the table, one of the staff members introduced herself. "Hi! My name is Katie. Welcome to immersion. We are so excited you are here!" she said. Katie asked for my name and I jokingly replied, "Big Sexy." She laughed and told me she didn't see that name on the list. I gave her my real name and she handed me my nametag and a green swag bag full of immersion-related gifts. She then asked if she could take my picture and I agreed to her request.

Michael received his nametag and bag of goodies, and then the two of us headed toward the elevator. I began digging through my swag bag as we waited by the elevator doors. I noticed a black exercise mat and a huge immersion workbook. The workbook featured information on the scheduled speakers, copies of the slides that would be used during lectures, as well as space to take notes. The bag also contained a water bottle and a bunch of healthy food samples. Michael and I agreed the bag was a nice surprise.

After dropping off our suitcases in our room, we headed downstairs to the oceanfront lawn for the scheduled welcome reception. Michael made small talk in the elevator. I could sense he was as nervous as I was. As the elevator doors opened to the magnificent hotel lobby, I could see lots of people carrying their newly issued goodie bags. All at once it appeared as though the entire resort was full of people attending the immersion program. There had to have been almost one hundred and fifty people taking part in the retreat. I took a deep breath, and then Michael and I headed out back to the reception area.

As we walked through the hotel's rear exit, it became immediately apparent that this was no fat camp. Yes, there were some people in the crowd who were definitely overweight, but there were many who looked trim and even fit. We headed over to the appetizer tables and were blown away by how colorful everything was. The combination of different foods really looked like an edible rainbow. Given my lifestyle, I had never really seen anything quite like it before. There were pineapple slices, berries of all kinds, melon wedges, cucumber slices, carrot sticks, and even avocados. Dozens of people were taking pictures of the spread with their cell phones. It was obvious that the collective first impression of immersion was pure astonishment.

I don't know if it was the fact that I was standing less than fifty yards from the ocean or that the appetizers were almost too beautiful to eat, but I suddenly experienced an overwhelming feeling of gratitude for the opportunity I'd been given. Without question, I knew I was exactly where I was supposed to be.

MEETING DR. STOLL

After a few minutes of mingling with some of my fellow immersion-ists at one of the tables on the lawn, I noticed a tall, slim man with dark hair making his way through the crowd. I could hear people starting to whisper that this was Dr. Stoll. As I watched him intro-duce himself to people, I happened to notice a little girl of around three years old walking around the reception area out of the corner of my eye.

I must admit, I was surprised to see such a young child there. I soon realized there wasn't just one child present but several. They ranged in age from two years old to fifteen. I watched in amazement as the little girl walked up to Dr. Stoll as he was talking to someone. The doctor immediately stopped what he was doing and gave her his full attention. After a brief exchange, the young girl made her way over to one of the teenagers, who picked her up.

That's when it hit me: Dr. Stoll had brought his family to immer-sion. Instead of keeping them separated from our group, however, as though they were on vacation, he had his family mingle with everyone in the program. I was left speechless, to be honest, and impressed. I had expected immersion to be something akin to going to see my own doctor, which was typically a cold and impersonal affair. It seemed this would be a rather different experience.

Having been preoccupied with this surprising sight, I hadn't noticed Dr. Stoll making his way over to me. I looked up and saw him standing right in front me. "Hi! I am Doctor Scott Stoll. I am so glad you are here," he said, extending his hand to shake mine. As I shook his hand and introduced myself, I got the feeling this doctor wasn't like any I had ever met. He seemed very genuine as he spoke to me. He came across as both humble and approachable. I immediately felt at ease as we began to chat. He told me he was looking forward to getting to know me over the next week, and then he excused himself and continued to make his way through the group of attendees.

As I stood there feeling the Florida sun on my face, nothing was as I thought it would be. I began to feel truly excited for what was to

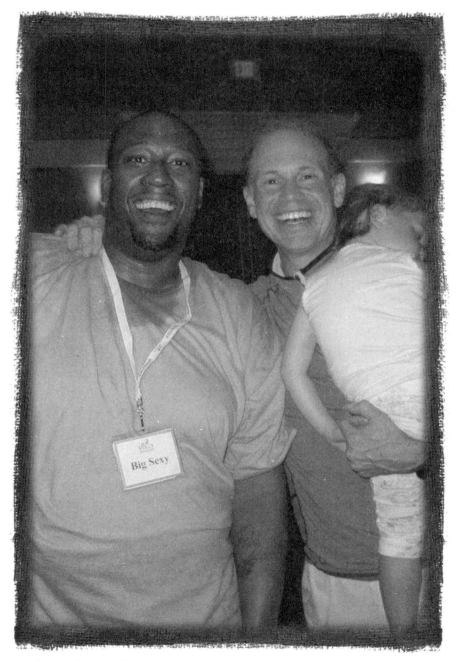

Milan and Dr. Stoll, the creator of the program that would change his life.

come. I was ready to become fully immersed, so I continued to introduce myself to other immersionists.

After spending about forty-five minutes at the welcome reception, I decided to return to my room to freshen up before the welcome dinner that evening. Michael stayed behind to chat with the others a little more while I went upstairs. As soon as I entered my room, I grabbed the phone to call my wife. I wanted to tell her all about my experience thus far. We talked about the resort and my meeting Dr. Stoll. She, too, was quite surprised to hear that the doctor had brought his entire family to the retreat. I told her I would call her later, and then we said our good-byes.

I took a quick shower, changed clothes, and headed back downstairs to the welcome dinner. The large banquet hall was stunning. There were identical buffet lines set up on each side of the room. Down the middle of the room were many large round dining tables set with white table linens and very creative centerpieces. At one end of the room there stood a wall of windows facing the ocean. The room looked more like a fine dining restaurant than a health retreat cafeteria.

I reached for a dish and got in line. The dinner buffet was just as impressive as the spread at the welcome reception had been. There were so many choices. I thought eating plant-based dishes meant eating bland, tasteless food. I had no idea healthy food could be so appetizing. I walked the buffet line and loaded up my plate.

I found numerous items with which to make a hearty salad. Frankly, there were items I had never personally considered putting on a salad—options such as black beans, chickpeas, and edamame beans. The dressing choices were eye-opening as well. I didn't know you could make ranch salad dressing without milk and have it actually taste like ranch salad dressing. I made my salad so big that I had to get a second plate for other types of food. Farther down the buffet line I saw vegan lasagna and ricotta. I couldn't believe this was what healthy eating could be like.

I took a seat at an empty dining table by the wall of windows. My roommate, Michael, soon spotted me and joined me. Before long, our table filled up with a group of people most would have considered a ragtag bunch. In addition to Michael, the table included José, a young Spanish-speaking African-American kid from Pennsylvania by way of the Dominican Republic; Madeline, an extremely creative Caucasian woman from Boston; Angela, an African-American woman with a genuineness I admired; Connie, a Caucasian woman who worked as a chef in New York; Alex, a five-foot-tall Hispanic woman from Virginia Beach with a great, outgoing personality; Gail, an older Hispanic woman who was always laughing and smiling; Monica, an older Caucasian woman from Chicago who had a very nice camera and loved to use it; and finally Rachel, an engaging Asian woman from Washington, D.C.

After dinner, our little group decided to meet on the beach to watch the sun set. Once nature's spectacular display had ended, we made our way to the back patio immediately outside the banquet hall. We told stories about our backgrounds and laughed a lot. Before we knew it, it was midnight. Knowing we had to get up early the next morning, we all retired to our respective rooms.

$\mathscr{D}$r. Stoll's Story

As we exited the hotel and walked toward the immersion program's oceanfront welcome reception, my wife, six children, and I saw the attendees—whom we called "immersionists"—gathered together, some seated at the tables on the lawn, some standing, and all representing a wide variety of states from across the country. There were even a few people from other countries.

I knew these people came from every walk of life based on the questionnaires they had filled out in advance, but they all had one common goal: reclaiming lost health. My wife, Kristen, and I had decided to make the immersion program a family project from the very beginning. This time every member of our family (Faith, age two; Elijah, age five; Joyous, age seven; Samuel, age nine; Gabriel, age eleven, and Dawson, age fifteen) would participate in the retreat and even take part in a family cooking presentation.

We felt it was important for participants to see enthusiastic children who were excited about the food they were eating and happy to fill their plates with vegetables at every meal. We knew that watching our kids eat well would help rid the attendees of the outdated mindset that children don't like vegetables or wouldn't be happy maintaining a proper diet. Having an actual example of healthy and contented children throughout the week always seemed to spark new outlooks in the immersionists, motivating them to go home and influence their own children in positive ways.

My wife and I visited each of the small groups gathered around the outdoor reception tables and warmly welcomed them to immersion. From the looks on many of the attendees' faces, I could tell they had a number of familiar questions on their minds: Is this really the answer? Can I do this? Will I be able to overcome my diseases and weight issues and feel better? What have I gotten myself into this time?

I approached one table and shook hands with a man who introduced himself as Milan Ross. "But you can call me Big Sexy," he said with a laugh as he pointed to his nametag and flashed a dynamic, contagious smile. I could tell this was going to be a fun and unique immersion because of his big personality and infectious laughter, but I also quietly prayed that Milan would find true freedom and joy during the week.

I considered the idea that the adoption of a nickname often suggests that the person using it is not comfortable with his or her actual self, and so has created an alter ego to escape possible pain, fear, guilt, or insecurity. As I walked away from Milan's table, I thought there might be something hidden behind his chuckles and smiles that would hopefully be revealed during immersion— something that would be the key to his freedom.

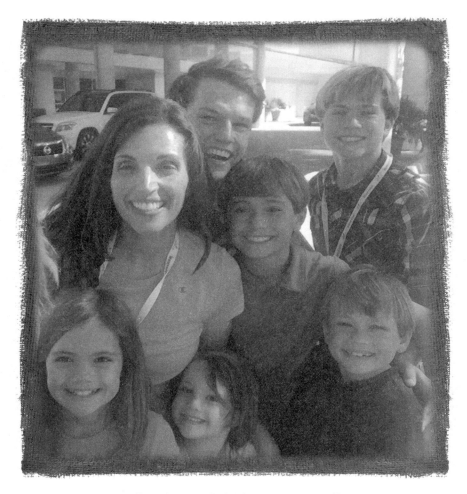

Kristen Stoll and the Stoll children arriving at the retreat.

Later that evening, with the sun getting low over the Gulf of Mexico, we all found ourselves in the banquet hall for our first dinner together. The buffet was beautifully arranged with a vibrant salad station, an array of spices, delicious cooked dishes, and a large bowl of hearty black bean soup. It was the first whole meal of the week, and for some it was the first healthy meal in decades.

At the outset of each immersion program, I always give a welcome speech after the first dinner. This speech outlines the expectations for the week, explains what happens to the human body once it starts consuming nutritious food, and casts a vision for a future in which healthy eating has become the cornerstone of life's foundation. I got the group's attention and began to speak.

Good evening, and welcome to health immersion. This entire retreat is an amazing opportunity to pull back from the time-consuming affairs of daily life, reevaluate how you have been living and the decisions that have brought you here today, and, perhaps for the first time, truly consider where you are going and how the food you eat today will directly influence the type of life you will live in the future.

Food is exceedingly powerful—more powerful than you might have thought. In modern Western culture, the concept of food has been reduced to calories, weight management, single nutrients, pleasure, convenience, necessity, and entertainment. Food means so much more, however, and I sincerely hope by the end of this retreat you will have begun to see how powerful, foundational, and beautiful healthy food can be.

Food is life; you can live only forty days without food. Food is health; the right food has the power to prevent, suspend, or reverse the majority of common diseases facing people today. Food choices are an inheritance; the food you eat today influences your DNA in just a few hours after eating it, and the effects of your choices extend two generations after you.

Your food choices impact the way you spend your money, choose your friends, and follow traditions. They can indirectly influence the strength of your marriage and family, alter your career and future plans, affect your savings, change your mood, modify your ability to think and reason, and ultimately transform opportunities for you to express and share your unique gifts with the world.

Finally, your food choices directly impact your broader relationships with your community, nation, and world. The breadth and depth of the influence of food are truly astounding, and this week I will walk you through a comprehensive review of scientific evidence that demonstrates the ways in which the right food choices can optimize every aspect of your body and life. This immersion will bring new inspiration and meaning to your meals as you begin to eat with new awareness, enlightenment, hope, and joy.

The really good news is that the food choices that bring newfound vitality and healing also happen to be delicious. Healthy food should be absolutely great. You are not required to settle for less. You won't be sacrificing taste for health here. This week you will experience food in a way that will be satisfying to your tongue and fulfilling to your body.

Realize that the power of food can influence you to do things you might normally consider outrageous. Case in point, a few years ago, at the end of an immersion week, a participant shared with us the fact that she had traveled to the retreat with a dozen of her favorite donuts. She had thought she would not be able to make it through the week without a dozen of her "glazed friends" supporting her throughout the process, but after my opening speech, she had begun to feel somewhat optimistic and decided she would leave the donuts in her luggage that night, and maybe eat one the next day.

According to this attendee, during the first day of lectures, hope had begun to rise up within her, causing her to throw the donuts away. She had put the box of donuts into one of the trash receptacles in the lobby that first afternoon, but her struggle against the power of the donuts had not ended. The woman told us that every time she would walk by that trash can on her way to and from her room, she would be extremely tempted to reach inside the can and pull out a donut! Lingering by the garbage, she would fight the urge for one quick reach and grab, restrained only by her fear that someone might come along and find her with her hand in the trash or glazed sugar on her lips. She had felt no uncertain relief after the receptacle had been emptied a few days later.

Aside from telling this amusing anecdote for your enjoyment, I'm relating this woman's story because it shows that she gained freedom and authority in her life over food during the week of immersion. As such, she was able to share this truth with the group. The story is a celebration of victory. It highlights how unhealthy food can consume your thoughts, weaken your will, and encourage you to reach harmful decisions. During immersion it is very common to have dreams about food, find yourself fantasizing about your favorite junk food, create detailed defenses of your favorite comfort foods, or even develop elaborate plans to acquire these foods in secret!

Eliminating unhealthy items from your diet, in fact, may result in potent physical withdrawal symptoms. This week you may experience acute headaches, nausea, clouded thoughts, diarrhea or constipation, stomach discomfort, generalized aches and pains, rashes, bad breath, or gas. You may also feel extreme fatigue to the point where you cannot keep your eyes open during lectures. The good news is that in approximately three to four days these withdrawal symptoms will pass and you will feel better than you have in decades. Experiencing these conditions is a very palpable reminder of the power of unhealthy food and its troublesome effects on your body.

By the end of immersion, most people comment that they can't remember a time when they felt so clear, energetic, strong, and pain-free. The short-term discomfort of withdrawal over the next couple of days is pain with purpose, so press on. You will be free from the bondage of cravings, food addiction, and toxic hunger before you know it.

During the withdrawal process, you must drink lots of water—six to eight glasses a day—and don't give in to the temptation to eat junk food. You can move past such enticement by getting enough rest, going for walks, calling friends for support, praying, relaxing, or standing on the declaration that you are stepping into freedom.

Tomorrow, the first full day of your new lifestyle begins. The lectures will help you understand the mindsets and thoughts that keep you bound to unhealthy food and lead you down a path toward diet-related diseases. You will begin to replace old thoughts with new, empowering beliefs that naturally produce good choices and a sustainable healthy lifestyle. Before bed, I would like you to recite the following affirmation aloud as many times as necessary until you are able to say it with conviction.

Today I declare I can change, and will be successful, and my past will not influence my success this week.

I believe I am able to change and will have all the resources I need to make this change.

I choose to receive new information gratefully and engage in healthy activities joyfully every day.

I am thankful for the opportunity to change, the freedom to choose, the hope of a new day, and the love of family and friends.

Your words have power. By reciting positive messages aloud, you can begin to shift your beliefs and empower your will.

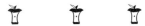

After giving this welcome speech to the attendees of the immersion program, I made one request of the group for that night, as I always do. I asked each of them to go for a relaxing walk on the beach and then get a restful night's sleep. Tomorrow would truly be a new day.

DAY
TWO

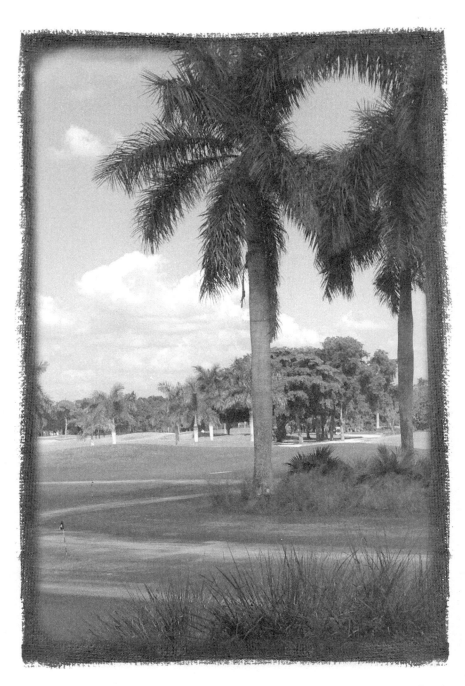

The view from the hotel patio, a popular meeting spot for Milan's immersion family.

Milan's Story

Unlike my experience the day before, I awoke with a positive attitude on the morning of my second day at the retreat. Unfortunately, it lasted only until I realized I would not be having my usual eight shots of espresso to start my day. My normal routine was to get out of bed and make myself an iced caramel macchiato with four shots of espresso. I would drink that down every morning as I got ready for work, and then I would make myself a second one to take with me on the drive.

It was shortly after 6 AM. I looked around my hotel room and noticed the coffee pot, but there was no coffee to be found anywhere. It occurred to me that perhaps this was not an oversight by the maid service. A quick call to the front desk confirmed my suspicion that there would not be any kind of caffeine permitted during this seven-day immersion.

I don't know why, but I had never thought of the possibility of not having access to things like caffeine, salt, sugar, or oil while at immersion. I suppose I should have expected such restrictions. I was on a health retreat, after all. On the surface, the notion of letting go of these items for one week may not sound terribly stressful, but I was a bit concerned about how I would function without my daily doses of coffee.

A quick peek at the agenda for the week reminded me that I needed to get going. I had been scheduled to have blood work done in about an hour. During the welcome dinner the night before, we had been informed that we would each have blood drawn and measurements taken before breakfast. Apparently, when you switch to a plant-based diet of whole food, your body can change pretty quickly, so it's important to monitor things closely in case certain medications need to be adjusted or stopped altogether. This initial blood test was meant to present an accurate picture of my health status before beginning immersion. It would later be compared to blood work performed on the final day of the program.

By the time I got out of the shower, my roommate, Michael, had already left to get his blood drawn, so I took a moment to phone Iris and check in. Despite it being two hours earlier in Colorado, I knew she wanted me to call. We talked about all the people I had met the night before. I told her how we had all hung out on the patio, chatting and getting to know each other. I explained how diverse the group was. There were both young and old people at the retreat, and they seemed to come from a wide array of cultures. For all the ways in which we were different, though, we all seemed to be connected by one thing: the need to improve ourselves. Even those who appeared to be healthy on the outside had medical conditions that required attention.

As I checked in with the immersion staff downstairs to get my blood work done, one of the staff members, Tom, approached me and asked if there was a problem with my nametag. At first I wasn't sure what he was talking about, but I soon remembered and jokingly told him my nametag was incorrect. "It should actually say 'Big Sexy,'" I said. He laughed and told me one of the other staff members had said I needed a new one, so he had made it for me.

Tom handed me my new nametag, which said "Big Sexy," of course. I asked him if I was actually allowed to wear the joke nametag, and he said yes, so I tucked it into my lanyard to display. One side of my lanyard showed my real name, Milan Ross, while the other side read "Big Sexy." I didn't know it at the time, but that nickname would end up sticking. Before the week ended, everyone knew me by that moniker, including hotel staff and program staff.

After being poked and prodded for about an hour, it was time for breakfast. I headed to the hotel banquet hall and made myself a nice big bowl of steel-cut oatmeal with fresh blackberries. I also got some tofu scramble, which kind of looked like scrambled eggs to me. My job at Whole Foods had introduced me to a new world of health foods, but knowing of them and actually eating them were two different things. Since coffee was not an option, I decided to try one of the green smoothies available. After filling my plate to capacity, I again made my way over to my table from the night before. Michael had already saved me a spot.

While sitting down to breakfast, Michael and I began discussing our concerns over what the results of our health tests might say. After a while, our conversation turned to which exercise class we would attend after our morning meal. As part of the immersion process, all participants were required to attend one exercise class each day. We noticed several from which to choose. No matter your fitness level, there was a class available to you.

As we discussed the many choices, a few of our new friends from the night before joined us at the table. We all began talking about our options and finally agreed to take the "Visibly Fit" class run by instructor Wendie Pett at 11 AM. After finishing up our breakfasts and chatting leisurely for a while longer, we all headed outside to the Tower Lawn for the class. The location had gotten its name from a huge plot of well-manicured grass that had been strategically designed between two of the hotel's beachfront towers. Needless to say, the view was breathtaking. During the exercise session, we even got to see dolphins swim by as we learned all about how our bodies could be our gyms.

Wendie taught us a method of exercise that didn't require a gym or gym equipment. When the class began, I was a bit skeptical, but she walked us through different movements that required us to create tension in our muscles using only natural muscle contractions. I could feel my body beginning to tire. I had chosen Wendie's class because I'd thought it would be the easiest, but I quickly realized these low-impact exercises were pretty tough—and very effective. By the time class was over, I was exhausted. I felt as though I had been lifting weights in a gym.

THE FIRST LECTURE

After the morning exercise class, Michael and I headed back to our room to freshen up. We had about an hour and a half to go before the first lecture of the day, which was being held at 1:45 PM. While lectures would begin at an earlier time on the remaining days, today's lecture had been scheduled to take place after lunch due to all the participants getting blood work done that morning. Michael told me he would be going back to the main floor shortly, but I was beginning to feel the effects of having skipped my morning coffee, so I decided to use this free time to take a quick nap. I was hoping it would help ease the dull headache that was quickly making its presence known.

My nap lasted about forty-five minutes, after which I headed back downstairs to eat lunch. I walked into the banquet hall and was pleasantly surprised by the choices I found. I grabbed a salad plate and made a big salad, topping it with all kinds of yummy items, and then I took another plate and walked quickly over to the veggie wraps. They looked fantastic—overflowing with peppers, onions, squash, and bean sprouts. I took a couple of wraps and continued down the buffet line.

Next I came upon what looked like a big pot of collard greens. I was familiar with this type of greens, so I spooned a big helping onto my plate and doused it with hot sauce. Farther down the buffet line, I began to read the menu cards placed in front of each food item. To my surprise, I saw ratatouille. I had eaten this dish many times before, so I was excited to try this new, healthier version. I rounded out my lunch with a cup of three-bean salad and pumpkin seeds, and then headed to my usual table in front of the wall of windows.

Not long after I had taken my seat, Michael sat down to join me. We weren't the only two people at the table for long, as pretty soon our other new friends found us. We all discussed how awesome the food was proving to be at the retreat. We also recognized the fact that some of us were starting to feel the effects of not drinking coffee. It wasn't just me; everyone seemed to be dragging a bit and fighting off a headache. Shortly after 1:30 PM, we left the banquet hall and made our collective way to the ballroom for our first lecture. It was time to learn what Dr. Stoll's Immersion program was all about from the man himself.

I entered the ballroom, grabbed myself a cup of caffeine-free herbal tea, and took a seat at the rear of the room. Michael chose a seat at the front on the opposite side of the room. Seating had been arranged in a classroom configuration. There were rows of long tables with multiple chairs at each one, all lined up perfectly, and a wide center aisle separating the two sides of the room. A pen and notepad lay waiting at each seat. Hanging at the front of the room was a large "Dr. Stoll's Immersion" banner, and a projection screen and podium stood onstage. To the rear of the room, where the entrance was located, there were two tables that had been set up on either side of the doors. They had herbal teas and fruit-infused waters for the guests. Grouped in the back corner, I couldn't help but notice a film crew with lots of camera equipment.

The room filled up rather quickly, and Tom, the staff member who had given me my new nametag, got up to address the crowd. He formally introduced Dr. Stoll, Dr. Stoll's family, and the rest of the immersion team, which consisted of three physical trainers, three health coaches, a nurse, and a physician. Dr. Stoll then described what attendees should expect from the retreat and outlined the best way to begin our transformations. As Dr. Stoll walked us through the program's intentions and methods, I began to get excited about the upcoming week. I grabbed the pen and notepad in front of me and began writing down the highlights of the speech. I was particularly taken by a concept Dr. Stoll called the "why," which he described as the big picture of a person's life, the vision that reveals the foundations of an individual's lifestyle and habits. I was fascinated by the idea of seeing my life from a new perspective and understanding my "why." If I could view the roots of my mindset and behavior more clearly, perhaps I could also untangle myself from them.

After about an hour or so, Tom stepped up to the microphone to announce a ten-minute break before the second lecture, which would feature guest speaker Dr. Sean Stephenson. During the break, many of the attendees gathered on the huge patio out back, which overlooked the hotel's world-class golf course. We all chatted about how thrilling it was to have the first lecture behind us. Until now, things had been fairly easy. Judging from the large workbook we had received in our swag bags the day before, however, the retreat would be a constant education from here on out. Before we knew it, the break was almost over, so we headed back to the ballroom.

As I returned to my seat, I saw a man of small stature in a wheelchair onstage. It was Dr. Sean Stephenson. I leafed through my workbook to find his biographical material, the content of which made me very interested to hear him speak. According to the information provided, Dr. Stephenson was not expected to survive long after birth due to a rare bone disorder, *osteogenesis imperfecta,* which stunts growth and causes bones to become very fragile. In spite of numerous challenges, however, he went on to become a doctor of clinical hypnotherapy, an internationally published author, and one of the leading motivational speakers in the world.

I learned that Dr. Stephenson had spoken in front of virtually everyone, from President Bill Clinton to His Holiness the Dalai Lama. He had appeared on top-rated national television shows such as *The Oprah Winfrey Show,* and had even had a network special about his life air on the Biography Channel. He would also go on to give a TEDx Talk at Ironwood State Prison in Blythe, California. I felt fortunate to be in the audience for his speech, which was titled "Time to Stand."

He began his lecture by sharing his personal story, which dealt with the significant physical and mental difficulties he had faced throughout his life. According to Dr. Stephenson, these trials and tribulations formed his "why," referring to the concept Dr. Stoll had mentioned earlier. Distilling this idea into one simple statement, Dr. Stephenson defined the "why" as the reason a person thought his or her life was the way it was. He then said he would like to ask five people to stand up and individually share his or her "why." I remember thinking there was no way I was going to get up and share something so personal with a room full of strangers. He began to pick people randomly from the audience. The first four were chosen—and then he pointed to me. I was to be the fifth.

THE HEAVIEST WEIGHT

I made my way to the microphone, which had been placed not onstage but in the aisle at the center of the room. I stood last in line behind the four other attendees who had been picked, my heart racing as I waited for my turn to speak. I thought about the question Dr. Stephenson had posed, and listened somewhat distractedly to the others as they shared their answers. I was attempting to figure out what exactly I thought my "why" was.

I had never given this question much thought. Things in my life were the way they were, I thought, because that's just how life works. I had never considered the fact that maybe there was something bigger lying just beneath the surface. Finally, it was my time to speak.

I approached the microphone and introduced myself. "Hi, my name is Milan," I said, as I nervously tried to adjust the microphone stand to my six-foot-four height. What I shared next surprised even me. I began to explain to this room full of strangers what my "why" was. Until then, I hadn't understood what my "why" was at all, actually. The answer came to me only after I had been asked the question directly, which had forced me to stop and think about it. This moment would prove to be a pivotal one in my life.

I explained that I had been very close to my mother. Being the youngest of five children, you might think I didn't get much attention at home, but I never felt as though my mother wasn't there for me. During my early childhood, my mother even started a tradition with me for my birthday. Every year, my mother would wake me at the exact time I entered the world on the day of my birth: 3:03 AM. She would make herself a cup of coffee and make me a cup of hot chocolate with marshmallows. She would also make us toast with strawberry preserves on it. We would sit at our kitchen table, just the two of us, and talk about whatever I wanted to chat about. It was a magical time.

When I eventually moved out of my childhood home, my mother and I still kept our tradition. Mom would call me on my birthday every year at 3:03 AM. We would sit at our respective kitchen tables, have coffee and toast, and chat about life. This habit might sound strange, but it was something I looked forward to all year long.

As I got older, I began to wonder how my birthday tradition had started, so I asked my mother. She said she remembered lying in her hospital bed with me in her arms on the day I was born. She had spent hours talking to me. She said it felt as though she and I were the only two people awake in the entire world during those hours. She had created my birthday tradition to experience that feeling again—a few hours during which we were the only ones awake in the world. It was wonderful.

In the summer of 2003, however, everything changed. My mother and I ended up having a major disagreement. This argument caused a rift that would change my life. Even though I have kept a journal since childhood, I never wrote down what that fight was actually about. Now I can't even remember.

Both of us were pretty stubborn. This stubbornness made us go from talking practically every day to not at all. I had truly thought the standoff would end at some point, but before I knew it, weeks of silence had turned into months of silence. I told myself that by December 30, my birthday, this standoff would end. My mother would call, and we would move past the last six months and catch up on everything.

On the day before my birthday, I went to the grocery store to pick up what I would need for my traditional birthday phone call. I couldn't stop thinking about what it was going to be like when we spoke. By 2:45 AM I began getting everything ready. I put on a pot of water for coffee, and got my toaster out of the cupboard to make toast. By 3 AM I was sitting at my kitchen table with my coffee and toast, telephone in hand. By 3:10 AM I started growing concerned, but I told myself my mother's clock could be off by a few minutes, so I should just give it more time.

At some point around 3:45 AM, I realized my mother was not going to call. I remember sitting at my table in tears. I was hurt. I couldn't believe she would end our tradition. I never considered my role in what was happening. I was now angry, and at that moment vowed never to contact her again. Besides a brief encounter five days before my son was born, my mother and I never spoke to or saw each other again.

On September 3, 2008, my mother, Joanette Ross, died of cancer. All at once, my tomorrows and second chances were gone. I never got the chance to make things right with her.

As I spoke of my relationship with my mother I could feel my throat tighten and my voice begin to tremble, but I needed to continue. I admitted to the group that I couldn't even remember the reason for the original fight. I felt a tremendous amount of guilt. I realized I had wasted years being mad over something that clearly wasn't important enough to recall. I couldn't stop thinking of the fact that my mother had never met my son.

I finished sharing my story with everyone in the ballroom and tears began to flow freely down my face. I looked out at the crowd and it seemed as though the entire audience was crying with me. People began hugging me on the spot. Dr. Stephenson told me that he was sure my mother had forgiven me for my part in what had happened between us. He told me he could see how much I loved her, and he was certain she wanted me to go and live my life fully. It was okay to let go of the guilt.

To my surprise, the "why" Dr. Stephenson had asked us to speak about had been buried in my soul for years. Given that moment, it simply poured out of me. I had been unexpectedly relieved of the heaviest weight of all that day. In opening up to this group of near strangers, I was able to release all the shame and guilt of losing my mother long before cancer took her from this world.

THE CHANGE BEGINS

We had an hour of free time before dinner at 6:15 PM. I decided to use it to take a long walk on the beach. I wanted to take some time to process what had just occurred. I had never spoken of my mother to anyone besides my wife. I realized I had just stood in front of a room full of people I had just met and completely bared my soul. I was a little embarrassed but also comforted.

After my walk, I went to my room and called Iris to tell her what had happened. My eyes welled up with tears again as I spoke to her. When our phone call ended I remember sitting alone silently, feeling that something was now different, although I could not say exactly what.

I went down to dinner and quickly found lots of people coming up to me to let me know how much my story had touched them. I met Michael and the others from our unofficial group at our favorite dining table and we chatted about how immersion was proving to be unlike anything we had imagined. We were being challenged in ways none of us had expected.

REVELATIONS

Michael and I walked over to the ballroom shortly before 8 PM to see the final lecture of the day. Presented by Dr. Stoll, it was called "Wellness Navigation: Why You Need a GPS." In his speech, Dr. Stoll explained why fad diets never result in long-term success. I sat there thinking how it all made sense. If you change something simply to achieve a particular result and then return to your normal routine after that result has been achieved, you will inevitably undo your accomplishment. Basically, without making a lifestyle change, you shouldn't expect any transformation to last.

Dr. Stoll's lecture wrapped up around 9 PM, at which point Michael and I went out to the patio again, where we found our new friends José, Madeline, Angela, Connie, Alex, Gail, Monica, and Rachel had all had the same idea. We talked in a group about how impactful the day's sessions were. I admitted I was a bit embarrassed by the emotional moment I had experienced during Dr. Stephenson's lecture. The group quickly let me know I had nothing to be ashamed of. Then, one by one, everyone took turns sharing their own "whys."

Michael spoke about how he had always felt as though his mother loved his older brother more than she loved him. José shared the fact that he, too, had lost a parent to cancer. His father, who had been his role model, had actually died in his arms. Madeline, Angela, and Connie all talked about their lifelong struggles with weight and health issues. They had all dealt with self-esteem issues, which had lead to numerous problems in their relationships with the opposite sex. Alex had recently gotten divorced from an emotionally abusive spouse and was now a single mother of two young children. Gail had not allowed anyone to get close to her in quite some time, having given up searching for someone to love after years of disappointment. Monica had convinced herself that she didn't deserve love after her dad had walked out on the family. Finally, Rachel said her "why" was simply rooted in the fact that she was too lazy to get up off the couch and exercise.

By 11 PM, everyone was ready to call it a night. Michael and I returned to our room to get ready for bed. We chatted as each of us went through our nightly rituals. By 11:30 PM, it was lights out. I lay in bed thinking about all the individual "whys" of our little group. We had each experienced something that had put our lives on a common trajectory, one that we needed to change.

In all my years of dieting, I had never considered dealing with the emotional aspects of my condition. Getting healthy had always been about my appearance. I was starting to understand that the path to optimal health starts with the mind, not with the body, and it was this idea that occupied my thoughts as I began to drift off to sleep.

$\mathcal{D}$r. Stoll's Story

The melodic chirping of birds in the palm tree outside my window gently woke me to a new day in Naples. It had been a long night of tossing and turning, unfortunately, as I had injured my elbow playing football on the beach with my kids the day before. It had begun to swell overnight and was now looking a little puffed, besides being sore.

I knew my morning was going to be spent taking the immersion participants' blood samples, height and weight measurements, waist-to-hip ratios, and blood pressures. Recording this information now would give my team baselines to compare with the results of testing at the end of the week. I simply had to figure out a way to take a person's blood pressure without triggering the pain in my elbow. I modified my technique enough that it elicited minimal agony each time I reached out to pump the blood pressure cuff. By the end of the morning, though, I was relieved to be finished with the tests.

After a short rest, my family and I went downstairs to lunch, after which we headed to the hotel ballroom, where lectures would be held throughout the week. Once the immersion team had assembled onstage, my partner and head of operations, Tom, introduced me and my family to the audience. He then introduced our trainers, Wendie, B.J., and Allison; our health coaches, Malissa, Nicole, and Kim; our nurse, Lana; and our physician, Dr. McGee.

I stepped forward to give my first lecture of the retreat, opening my arms as wide as I could to welcome everyone and quickly reminding myself of my elbow injury. (I wouldn't do that again for a while.) I composed myself and began.

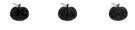

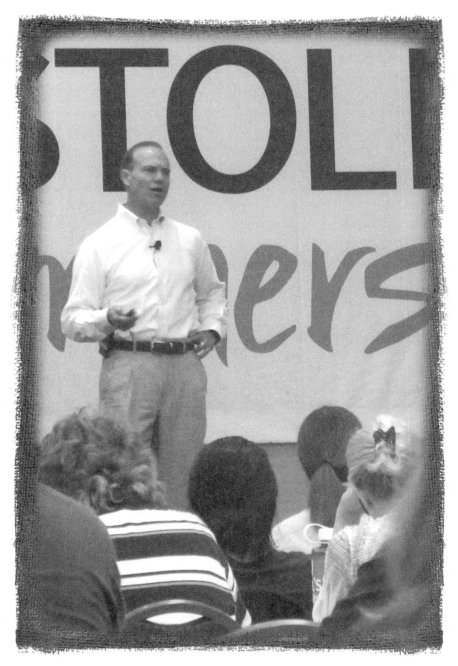

Dr. Stoll giving one of his scheduled lectures during immersion.

Good afternoon, and welcome to the first lecture of immersion. This week you will experience how quickly your body can begin to feel better, how fast inflammation can subside, how rapidly blood pressure and blood sugars can improve when you feed your body the right food, resolve sources of stress, and move more. You will also learn how food has the power to prevent, reverse, or suspend most common diseases, as well as influence your relationships, career, charity work, family life, and spirituality. Food is one of the most important foundations of your existence, and this week you will learn how to enjoy foods that enhance and expand every area of your being. You are in for an exciting adventure that can radically alter the trajectory and direction of your life. I will also introduce you to a few past immersionists who will share their amazing stories about their journeys to true health. These testimonials—which we call "reveals"—will inspire you and help you see what is possible when you make the change.

Now I want you to close your eyes. Take a big breath in through your nose, hold it a few seconds, and then slowly release it through your mouth. Repeat this routine one more time. Open your eyes and smile. Today is the first day of our lecture series, which has been designed to help you deconstruct some of your old mindsets, dated dietary and nutritional information, ineffective lifestyles, and emotional issues that may be keeping you unable to move forward, stuck with diseases that are reversible, medications that you shouldn't need, and beliefs that tell you change is not possible.

This week you will begin to create new ideas and mindsets, gain a fresh understanding of nutrition and food, and learn how to build a sustainably healthy life full of joy.

Imagine a large building with cream-colored marble floors, a polished stainless steel reception desk in the lobby, and two long upward escalators. It is early in the morning and the sun's rays are peeking through the building's three-story glass walls. The escalator is empty except for two sharply dressed business people, a man and woman, who are nearing the top, each with a coffee in one hand and a computer bag in the other. Suddenly and unexpectedly, the escalator comes to a jolting halt. Initially frustrated, they rummage through their bags for their phones and the woman exclaims, "I can't believe this. I am already late!" The man replies, "Don't worry, someone will come." Then he yells out, "Somebody, hello! There are two people stuck on an escalator. We need help. Would someone please do something?" He receives no response, hearing only his echo.

The two people begin to laugh at their unfortunate circumstance, resigned that they are stuck. They decide the only thing they can do is wait for help. After a long period of time, a voice calls out from ground level, "Hey! Don't worry! I will have you off that escalator in a second." They peer over the handrail and see a repairman on the other escalator riding up to the next level. "I'll get to the top of your escalator and fix it for you," he says.

Joyfully they watch the man and say to each other, "He said he can fix it. Now that's more like it." Suddenly, the escalator the repairman is riding grinds to a halt as well. The three people look at each other in disbelief. The man and woman give up hope, sit down on the escalator stairs just a few feet from the top, and wait for more help to arrive.

The question I would ask is: Are they really stuck?

I believe they are, actually. Even though they could simply walk up the remaining steps and reach their destination, they have a mindset that prevents them from seeing this solution. They have become dependent on outside forces to solve their problem. Sound familiar?

Of course, it is absurd to believe you might get stuck on an escalator. But if you are honest with yourself, and begin to look around, you will see many people who feel stuck in circumstances not unlike a broken-down escalator—people who have given up. These people share a certain attitude that blinds them to the very clear solution to any type of out-of-order escalator, which is to walk to the top!

Through many years of working with people at these immersions and in my own medical practice, I have found that when someone is "stuck" in regard to a health challenge, many times it is a problematic mindset that prevents recognition of what is actually a very clear solution. Before anyone can move forward positively, his or her mindset must change.

Here is the key principle to remember from today's lecture: Sustainable health begins and ends in your thoughts, beliefs, and emotions. The first and most important step in your health transformation is often the one that is overlooked because you want to skip ahead to tangible actions. "Just tell me what to do," you ask. Rarely does anyone say, "Help me know what to think, believe, and feel, so I can make a lasting change."

Thoughts, beliefs, and emotions before actions. "Be" before "do." Remember that you are a human being, not a human doing. Our culture has pressed all of us into a mode of doing—doing more with less is celebrated as success. The doing is important, of course, but it must follow a change in thoughts, beliefs, and emotions. This is the reason so many diets fail. They are built primarily on doing instead of being. The fact is that what you do occurs as a result of your thoughts, beliefs, and emotions, so it is only logical to start by addressing your state of being first when making a change in lifestyle. The doing part will follow.

Your actions and habits are the visible effects of your mindset. When these are in alignment, change is inevitable, effortless, and joyful. There are people whose stories inspire us to change ourselves, give us hope, and allow us to see the possibilities. Their outward changes are evidence of equally powerful inward changes. You will meet two such people later this week.

Unfortunately, some people, when inspired by a person who has made a positive transformation, may rush to action too soon, wanting to do whatever that person did to achieve success. In doing so, they frequently miss the change in mindset that brought about and sustained success. Often, these less tangible aspects of an individual's change are not mentioned or highlighted in any health books, videos, or speeches, which tend to focus on the observable steps of health programs.

Think of the connection between your mindset and your health like this: The routines adopted in a healthy lifestyle, such as exercising regularly and eating the right foods every day, are like a car and your mindset is like the fuel for that car. Sure, even if the car doesn't have any gas in it, you could push it down the road through pure determination—but only a short distance. Before long, your legs and lungs would be burning and you would begin to slump down on the bumper, frustrated and tired. But fill up the tank with high-octane fuel—the right thoughts, beliefs, and emotions—and the vehicle will leap to life and carry you wherever you want to go effortlessly. In other words, you can work out and eat healthfully all you want, but without the right mindset fueling these changes, you may always feel as though you are struggling.

This week I am going to help you fill up your tank with the right mindset, one that will help bring energy, health, and joy to your life.

THE GREATEST GIFT

The best way to start your transformation is to take stock of some of the gifts life has given to you. When you take advantage of these gifts each day, your thoughts, beliefs, and emotions will change.

The most important gift in life holds more power than you might think, and is often overlooked and squandered, but is actually the key to your future and well-being. The way you use it can dramatically affect your life and the lives of people around you and echo through generations.

So, what is this amazing gift that is so valuable and important to your present life and future? It is the gift of choice. Right now you have the power to choose what to think, believe, and feel. You can decide what to eat, what not to eat, to hate or to love, to embrace stress or to let it go, to hold on to anger and bitterness or to forgive, to be dissatisfied or to be grateful, to frown or to smile. And these are just a few of the choices within your ability.

From the moment you open your eyes in the morning, you make choices. I don't want you ever to forget that you have been blessed with this power. The combination of choices made today results in the reality of your tomorrow. You can redirect your life no matter where you are, right now, simply by making a different choice to point yourself in the right direction.

One choice added upon another creates your future. A good choice today added to a better choice tomorrow and so forth is a recipe for permanent change. The more positive choices you make, the more you accelerate change, so that before you know it the accumulation of good choices becomes a new lifestyle, leaving you wondering exactly when you became this new person.

Numerous factors may try to influence your power to choose and stop your change. Your emotions, beliefs, personal history, and perceived identity can manipulate your choices positively or negatively. You may not even realize that your decisions are being swayed by your overall mindset until someone brings this fact to your attention.

Beyond your mindset, external forces such as finances, work and living environments, people, cultural beliefs, marketing, and societal values may attempt to direct your choices, sometimes at your expense. For example, advertisements can influence you with appeals that touch upon perceived needs, desires, or deficits, providing rationales for decisions they would like you to make. One particular tobacco ad once boldly stated, "Give your throat a vacation; smoke a fresh cigarette." A certain soda ad has claimed the drink to be "happiness in a bottle." Can you see how these ads are merely trying to manipulate your choices in order to separate you from your money regardless of the negative health effects these products can have?

Before you buy that next sweet treat or salty snack, stop and ask yourself, "Why would I make this choice right now, what is my motivation, and how is the marketing of this product attempting to influence my decision?" Asking these questions is a great way to hit the pause button and gain some perspective and control. During this pause, remind yourself that you are, in fact, in control. You have the power to decide, and you are going to make the best possible choice.

Over the next week, I will explain in detail how your emotions and even food can strongly influence the choices you make, but right now I simply want you to understand that, no matter how powerful the stimulus may be, you still have the final word in your life. You can choose to say "Yes" to healthy food and "No" to unhealthy food.

Take a big breath and believe you are powerful, not powerless, that you are ultimately in control of your destiny, and that with every "Yes" and "No," you write your future.

A NEW DAY

Can you recall a time in your life when you were blessed by a brilliant sunrise and it filled you with hope? Can you see that day in your mind's eye—the brilliant golden sun as it slowly rises in the sky? Can you feel the warm rays of the sun as they gently touch your skin? How did that sunrise make you feel? Hopeful, joyful, energized, enthusiastic, strong, and alive. Why did you feel that way? You were experiencing the gift of a new day.

The second great gift given to you every twenty-four hours is the promise of a new day. When paired with the power of choice, a new day is a great opportunity to shape your future.

How frequently do you awaken with a joyful, grateful attitude? Now, we all face those mornings when the alarm is rudely signaling the start of a new day, even though it seems as if we've just closed our eyes. Our first thoughts might drift to how tired we are; how worn down, stressed out, and burned out we are; how we are not sure how we are going to make it; how we feel out of control, fearful, uncertain, and hopeless. Consider for a moment how these first thoughts spill over and affect the day.

They set you up for a day of more problems, more frustration, more challenges—a real Charlie Brown day—as your thoughts determine your attitude, your attitude determines your actions, and your actions influence your relationships and opportunities. You will end up getting exactly what you unconsciously chose thanks to those early morning thoughts. You will create the difficult day you envisioned.

But let's imagine a different scenario, one that you choose. Tomorrow morning, when you wake up, recognize the amazing gift of a new day. Take a breath and feel the air fill your lungs. You have choices at your disposal, and you have the opportunity of a day ahead, even if it is full of challenges. The day is full of possibilities, and you have the power to shape your future throughout your waking life. Your future does not have to look like your yesterday because you can begin to make different choices, which will lead you to different outcomes.

Wake up and let go of your old mindset, which has you stuck. Let go of the belief that you cannot make lasting changes because you don't have the willpower to do so. Let go of the idea that you can't change because you are different and face more challenging circumstances than everyone else. Let go of the notion that life is just too difficult and you don't have enough inside you to deal with it. Let those old mindsets go. They are not helping you, and they will only give you more of the same. I know that is not what you want.

You can change your mindset right now to include gratitude, hope, forgiveness, and empowerment by realizing that you have the power to choose, and so have the ability to change.

Philosophers, theologians, and researchers have all pointed to gratitude as one of the most important human emotions that impacts well-being.[1,2] In a study of 186 heart failure patients, gratitude was associated with improved mood, fewer feelings of depression, less fatigue, better sleep, better management of cardiac function, and lower inflammatory markers.[3] Interestingly, a large trial that used antidepressant medication failed to impact many of these same measures in heart failure patients.[4] It is the conscious choice to be grateful that produces positive effects. The answer lies in the will, not in a pill.

But how do you begin to change your mindset? You develop a habit of waking up in the morning and listing things you are grateful for that day. Write them all down and keep them on your nightstand as a daily reminder. Even if you can only think of one thing to be grateful for, concentrate on your one blessing throughout the day. There is always something to be thankful for, and that is the fact that you have the opportunity to make choices every day.

Make a list of all your blessings, practice acts of kindness and prayers of gratitude, think of people you appreciate and tell them of your appreciation, or start a journal and write about gratitude every day. Always remember that you have the gift of a brand new day.

THE POWER OF WORDS

The third gift you've been given is your words. Words have the power to create or to tear down, to heal or to harm. Words written thousands of years ago still have the ability to influence people today, and words spoken to you or about you decades ago may still have a positive or negative effect on your life presently. We have all experienced conversations in our minds that are just as alive today as they were when they occurred so many years ago. Did you know that your words create ripples of influence when you speak? The words you speak to others, the words they speak to you, and the words you speak to yourself have enormous potential.

Every day, we use our words to converse with others and even with ourselves. Research estimates that humans talk to themselves thousands of times a day. What are you saying to yourself? Sadly, it has been estimated that 77 percent of daily self-talk is negative. We may talk negatively to ourselves as we recall arguments, think through challenges, regret the past, fear possible futures, or quietly judge ourselves.

The self-talk most common to this immersion retreat includes phrases such as "I can't," "I always fail," "It's too difficult," "I am different and it's harder for me," and "It will never happen." Be aware of these toxic ideas sneaking into your internal monologue and sabotaging your opportunity for success. They are lies, and as soon as you think them, you can say to yourself, "Why can't I?" You can say, "I cancel that last comment because I believe I can."

Cancel lies and replace them with empowering, hope-filled words: I can change, I will change, I enjoy change, I will succeed, I believe I have the ability to change, I am creative, I am capable, and I can overcome any challenge.

Research has shown that a healthy relationship has a positive-to-negative comment ratio of five to one. In other words, people in a healthy relationship utter five positive comments for every one negative comment. The first step in developing positive relationships, including your relationship with yourself, is to be aware of the words you are speaking. Listen to yourself and take inventory of your statements. Consider how you may inject positive sentiments into a situation using words of hope, truth, encouragement, strength, courage, love, peace, compliment, or kindness. Utter life-enhancing words as much as possible and soon they will become a regular part of your daily conversations.

If you become anxious or stuck, rather than slip into despair or condemnation, stop and ask yourself, "What can I do right now?" Use your power of choice to take a positive step instead of a negative one. If you are fearful, ask, "What am I afraid of right now?" You will usually find it is not a life-threatening fear, and then you can release it. Anxious and fearful thoughts and words are sure to come up this week as you encounter new foods, new ideas, and new situations, so replace problematic self-talk with fruitful words as soon as it arises.

Your goal this week and beyond is to think and speak words of life. Speak life-enhancing words to each other and to any other people you meet during the day. Look for opportunities to encourage, inspire, and offer hope, joy, peace, and kindness to others. And don't forget to speak kindly to yourself. Intentionally practice this new skill every morning and evening by consciously talking positively to yourself for a few minutes.

Speak words of life and put a positive spin on an old script you've been reading for years. Perhaps part of that old script is a bitter conversation you recall repeatedly, which stirs up anger. Approach that part of your script by stopping the story and offering that person forgiveness. You will experience an amazing sense of relief. You will have released tension and allowed healing of that wound, which had harmed you over and over throughout the years. Set yourself free by choosing to forgive.

The idea that forgiveness somehow lets the person being forgiven off the hook, that forgiving means justice will never be served, is the main driving force of a mindset that is stuck. By holding on to the anger, bitterness, and resentment associated with a prior situation, it is you who are paying the price right now. Choose to forgive. I know it is not easy, but when you forgive you will feel light and joyful. Peace will fill the space in which toxic emotions once resided.

YOUR "WHY"

Have you ever tried to build a puzzle without the picture on the box top? One thousand pieces on the table and no photo to give context or perspective would lead most of us to get up and walk away, no matter how optimistic the mindset. Failure would seem almost certain due to the lack of connection between the pieces and the whole.

Sustainable change similarly requires a look at the bigger picture of your life. It is a vision of your life that reveals the need for a health-promoting diet and overall lifestyle. The food you eat, the emotions you embrace, and your activities each day are the individual puzzle pieces that build your future. A clear vision of your life is the box top that gives each piece meaning, value, and importance.

I like to call this vision your "why." A powerful and motivating "why" in life will clarify the critical importance of your diet and catalyze the process of change. It can mean the difference between working hard to make a lifestyle change and hardly working at all. Once you clearly establish your "why," you will understand the purpose behind the food you eat every day, and you will be pulled forward into making healthy decisions by a strong current of purpose. Knowing your "why" causes a passionate pursuit of your vision, infused with commitment, dedication, persistence, perseverance, enthusiasm, joy, creativity, and determination.

So, do you have a powerful, motivating "why" in your life that will lead to a permanent change? During each immersion, we ask people to write down their "whys" on pieces of paper and tape them up on a designated wall of the lecture hall for others to read. We call this wall the "why wall," and it is meant to serve as a source of inspiration. Some "whys" I have seen include "to live a long healthy life for my children and grandchildren," "to be well enough to travel to a third-world country and help others in great need," "to start teaching others in my community how to be healthy," "to overcome my diseases and be free to pursue my travel dreams," and "to be the best I can be so that I may bless those I love every day."

In contrast, the diet industry focuses on the short-term. If you have ever dieted, you know that you may work very hard, sweating and enduring discomfort to lose weight, only to find the change is temporary. After months of painful dieting, sacrifice, and exercise to reach your goal weight, you celebrate and reward yourself by reaching for the sweets and treats that were forbidden during your diet.

Deprivation, starvation, and sacrifice used only to reach a short-term goal are not methods that result in long-term sustainable change. As time passes, they lead back to old patterns, led by food addictions and emotional eating habits. Without a greater vision, a bigger picture, the number on your scale will soon increase again.

Sustainable change is empowered by your "why," so part of your homework this week is to find the "why" in your life, if you don't know it yet. Spend some time contemplating this idea and talking about it with a trusted friend or mentor. Determining your "why" is a process that takes time, so hang in there and continue to search. You will be rewarded with an amazing vision of your life. Don't give up.

You may find you have several "whys" in life, and that is fine. They are simply additional reasons to make the best choices every day. Once you have your "why," write it down, find pictures to inspire you to reach your vision, and ask a friend to remind you of your purpose. Recalling your "why" is like refueling your gas tank on a long journey. It is absolutely necessary.

I leave you all today with an affirmation that encapsulates the ideas put forth in this lecture, which will form the bedrock of your change.

I declare that I will reclaim my power of choice.

I have been given the gift of choice and authority, and I will honor that gift and myself by making better choices today.

I will make healthy choices today and choose a brighter future.

I believe I can change and know that I will change.

Today I choose to live in gratitude and see the many blessings of this day.

Tomorrow I will awaken and be grateful from the moment I open my eyes to the moment I lay my head down to rest.

I choose to be grateful for my life and the lives of those who love me.

Today I will choose gratitude over discontentment, disappointment, and dissatisfaction, and set my mind on the aspects of my life that are a blessing and abundant.

I believe I am grateful. I feel grateful.

I choose to plant the seeds of well-spoken words so that others and I may enjoy the fruits of life.

I will avoid conversations that are judgmental and critical, and instead speak words that bless, encourage, and support others and myself.

In every conversation I will look for opportunities to bring life, healing, encouragement, and joy.

Today is a new day and my future is in my hands. Today I choose life.

Please enjoy the second lecture of the morning, which will be given by the amazing Sean Stephenson, and the rest of this beautiful day.

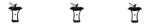

After the lecture, I was met by a number of people who had approached the stage with questions. A woman was holding a paper with some large letters written on it. I quickly recognized the penmanship of one of my younger children. I remembered I had noticed my two youngest walking from seat to seat in the ballroom just before the lecture, writing encouraging messages on the notepads of the immersionists. This participant was so grateful for the heartfelt encouragement. She said it had helped her so much that day that she was going to keep it, even though it had been a little misspelled. She turned the pad toward me and I read, "Your awsome, your an overcomer." The message had been misspelled, yes, but it was right on the mark when it came to heart and effort. Seeing it made for the perfect end to my lecture session that day.

DAY THREE

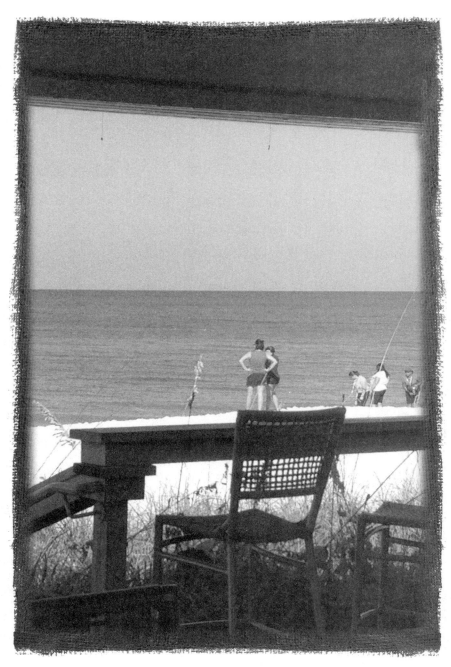

The ocean vista from the hotel's beachfront bar.

*M*ilan's Story

I awoke at 6:30 AM on Day Three to what I can describe only as a war being waged inside my body. My dull headache from the day before was now a brain-bending, nausea-inducing, vision-blurring storm. I was weak. I felt sluggish and unfocused. It was as if my body had decided to revolt against me for all the years of abuse to which I had subjected it. All I wanted to do was lie in bed all day, but a glance at the clock served as a reminder that I had about thirty minutes before morning exercise classes were scheduled to begin.

I kept thinking about how this is what heroin withdrawal must feel like. It felt as though I was trying to kick some kind of drug addiction. I was beginning to realize just how powerful a force food was in my life. It occurred to me that making a lifestyle change was definitely not going to be a walk in the park. I had assumed that eating healthy would make my body happy, but that certainly wasn't the case. My body didn't feel very happy. I kept telling myself the way I was feeling was a good thing because it meant my body was beginning to repair all the damage I had done to it. The old mantra "no pain, no gain" kept replaying in my mind.

After a quick shower, I got dressed, grabbed my green "Dr. Stoll's Immersion" water bottle, and both Michael and I made our way downstairs to join one of the morning fitness classes. On the elevator ride down, Michael confirmed that he, too, was feeling the effects of withdrawal. Since neither of us was feeling very good, we decided we would take the yoga class. I was hoping yoga would help me relax, which might make the discomfort I was experiencing a little easier to bear.

Michael and I settled into an open spot on the lawn. I positioned my exercise mat so that I had a clear view of both the class instructor and the ocean. The view really helped take my mind off the way I was feeling. Midway through the exercise class, I watched a group of dolphins swim by and wondered if they were the same ones I had seen the day before. I smiled at the wonder of nature and began to feel calm.

When the exercise class ended, Michael and I headed back to our room to drop off our exercise mats and grab our immersion workbooks. The yoga class seemed to have taken my mind off the symptoms I was experiencing, but as soon as it was over, I began to feel the full force of my pounding headache again. I needed to focus on something else, so I decided to take a moment to call home.

When Iris answered the phone, she could immediately tell I wasn't feeling well. I don't know if it was the sound of my voice that tipped her off or if she could simply sense I was not myself, but however she'd figured it out, my condition was giving her cause for concern. As I began to explain to her what was going on with me physically, Iris asked if I had spoken to any of the immersion staff about my symptoms. I told her I was planning on speaking with the medical team after breakfast. She made me promise to call her back and let her know how I was doing as soon as I could. With that, I told Iris I loved her, asked her to give Nigel a kiss for me, and said goodbye. Michael and I grabbed our things and headed downstairs to get some breakfast.

THIS TOO SHALL PASS

Upon entering the banquet hall, I could immediately see that Michael and I were not the only two people struggling through the withdrawal phase of immersion. As I glanced around the room, it was obvious everyone was feeling a bit off. Several people were sitting with their heads on their tables, while others just seemed to be staring aimlessly off into space. I heard numerous participants murmuring about headaches and fatigue. Their symptoms seemed to range from severe to mildly uncomfortable. No one appeared to be completely immune to the feelings of withdrawal. Just imagine an emergency room full of people waiting to see a doctor—without the bleeding, of course—and I think you'll get the picture.

I grabbed a green smoothie and fruit for breakfast. My headache had nauseated me and I couldn't eat any more than that. Michael and I took seats at our usual table, looked at the other immersionists sitting there, and recognized that everyone was feeling the same way. We barely spoke as we all tried desperately to eat. Finally, after about ten minutes of silence, someone blurted out, "Getting healthy sucks!" The table erupted in laughter and agreement.

As I finished my smoothie, I wondered if there was truly something better on the other side of all this discomfort I was experiencing. I can't deny that I considered using the next scheduled block of free time to walk to the closest convenient store and buy some snacks. Feelings of withdrawal from sugar, salt, and caffeine consumed my every moment, but somewhere in the back of my mind, I heard the whisper of a phrase my mother used to repeat often: This too shall pass.

Michael and I made a beeline for the ballroom shortly before the 9 AM lecture. I approached one of the immersion staff members and explained to her how I was feeling. To my surprise, she wasn't alarmed in the slightest. She told me my symptoms were completely normal and should pass in a day or two. I asked her for something to help with the headaches, she kindly gave me a packet of Tylenol, and off I went.

Michael and I took seats at the rear of the room and tried to prepare ourselves for the first lecture. A quick glance at the agenda reminded me that the first few lectures of the day would be given by Dr. Stoll himself. I was determined not to let my body ruin my opportunity to learn. Dr. Stoll was scheduled to discuss the concept of food addiction. I had never thought about food as truly addictive. For years I had thought my problem was merely that I lacked sufficient willpower and focus. He explained the notion of hunger in detail, what it does to the body and brain, and how to avoid unwanted reactions to hunger.

I was surprised to hear that even dairy products, which I'd thought were healthy choices, could have negative effects on digestion and were highly addictive. I was reminded of all the times I had been told as a child that I needed to drink milk in order to have strong bones. Being told that the dairy milk we drink was actually meant to take a baby calf and turn it into a two-thousand-pound cow in one year certainly adjusted my perspective. While it might have been obvious, I hadn't really considered the idea before. Although I was lactose intolerant, I still drank milk. I also gave it to my son because that's what I had been taught to drink as a child. I decided I would never consume cow's milk or give it to my son again.

As I listened to Dr. Stoll, I began to view hunger for what it truly was: a signal my brain uses to tell me it's time to eat. It sounded simple enough, but I now recognized that most people find it almost impossible to overcome their cravings for junk food when hunger occurs.

During the short break between Dr. Stoll's first lecture and his second, I exited the hotel to join a few of my fellow attendees who had congregated on the patio overlooking the golf course. Two immersion staff members were standing immediately outside the rear door, taking some of the participants' blood pressures. One of them signaled to me to come over and have a seat so she could take my reading. I sat down and she began checking my blood pressure.

I had had high blood pressure for as long as I could remember. In fact, I had been taking medication to help control my blood pressure at the time. On any normal day my blood pressure would have been 155 over 100, which is about what it was during my physical examination the day before. When the staff member completed my test, I asked her for my results. She quietly said, "100 over 77." With a puzzled look on my face, I asked her kindly to repeat what she said. "100 over 77," she said in a slightly louder voice. She could see I was confused. She asked me if everything was okay. I explained to her that something was wrong with her equipment because my blood pressure was always high, even with me taking medication to treat it.

The staff member explained to me that when you start eating healthy plant-based food, internal changes may occur quickly. Next, she reaffirmed what the other staff member who had given me Tylenol had said earlier. "Your headaches, nausea, and all the other symptoms you are experiencing should go away over the next day or so," she said. "Hang in there and you will be fine."

After the fifteen-minute break, I headed back to my seat for the next lecture. As I sat down next to Michael, my mind couldn't yet wrap itself around the information I'd just been given. I couldn't believe that in just a few short days, food had managed to do what my medication could not. My blood pressure was now in the normal range. After spending more than a decade and a half struggling to get my blood pressure under control, I wasn't showing signs of hypertension anymore. How could this be?

Dr. Stoll once again addressed the audience and began to talk about how to conquer hunger, food addiction, and cravings. Even though my head was still pounding, I was determined to pay attention. It was as if a light had been turned on inside me. Knowing healthy food had already begun to change me for the better really blew my mind. I had never thought of food as a vital part of my overall health. Yes, I was aware that humans need to eat to survive, but I'd never looked at food as medicine. *Why doesn't everyone know about this?* I thought. *Why aren't doctors telling their patients about this?*

In all the years my doctor had been treating my various conditions, she had never once mentioned a plant-based diet as a treatment option. She had told me I needed to lose weight, but she had never explained that eating a diet of mostly plants could help my body repair itself. I felt like an enormous secret was being kept from the people who really needed to know it. I paid close attention as Dr. Stoll laid out a very easy-to-follow list of practical steps to avoid the pitfalls of hunger. I would never think of cravings in the same way again.

PLANTS, NOT PILLS

Michael and I headed off to lunch after the morning's lectures. I took a detour and walked out to the beach to call my wife. Iris answered the phone and I immediately began to tell her about what had happened to my blood pressure. I explained how my reading was better on plants than it had been on pills. Iris listened intently. She remarked on my level of excitement and said she'd not heard me so enthusiastic in a very long time. I agreed with her. She asked me how my headache was, and I actually had to stop to think about it. It was there, but I could live with it. It was not going to ruin my day. After a few more minutes of conversation, I told Iris it was lunchtime and promised to call her back soon.

During lunch, Michael and I, along with all the rest of our new immersion family, sat and discussed our experiences at the retreat so far. There was lots of talk about how we were all feeling slightly ill, but we also chatted about the first two lectures of the day. Everyone seemed to be feeling some sort of overall transition. Moreover, we all felt hopeful, an emotion that had been absent from so many of our lives. I looked around the table and realized not one of us was going to leave immersion without the answers we needed.

Participants had begun to move beyond withdrawal. It wasn't that everyone was suddenly feeling better, but rather that we had started to realize that maybe this process was different. This program wasn't like any diet I had ever tried. I now know the reason for that: Immersion isn't a diet at all; it's a lifestyle change. Even though I was hurting, I knew I was getting stronger. My mind was getting stronger with each lecture. The more I learned, the more I realized I had a say in my health, both mentally and physically.

After lunch, everyone returned excitedly to the ballroom for Dr. Stoll's final lecture of the day. The idea of preventing and reversing disease with food opened my eyes to all the possibilities a plant-based diet presented. Dr. Stoll discussed how food could be used to stop the progression of many diseases, including heart disease and type 2 diabetes, and sometimes even reverse them. I couldn't believe what I was hearing. I began to understand that I didn't have to have high blood pressure simply because my dad, mother, and grandparents had suffered from hypertension. My heritage was not my destiny.

Throughout the speech, I found myself continually wondering if I had heard Dr. Stoll correctly. I even debated whether or not what he was saying was true. *Could it really be possible? Could I actually rid myself of all the health problems I had acquired?* As I sat there contemplating everything Dr. Stoll was saying, the one fact I couldn't escape was that my blood pressure had changed so quickly on the plant-based diet I had been following. This was a result even my medication struggled to accomplish. My belief in immersion and my resolve were growing stronger and stronger.

At the end of Dr. Stoll's final lecture of the day, he introduced Gail as the first reveal, the same Gail I knew as a member of my little ragtag meal club. Dr. Stoll explained that she had already gone through the program previously and had been asked to rejoin the retreat to show the new participants how she'd been doing since leaving her first seven-day immersion. You could have heard a pin drop as Gail made her way to the stage. Everyone listened intently as she shared her journey. We could not believe how far she had come. She had lost a total of thirty pounds, but what was more important than the weight loss was the new life she was now able to enjoy.

Gail told us how her health improvement had affected every aspect of her being. She could now do things with her grandkids that she never dreamed of doing before. Her happiness was evident. You could see it in the tears of joy that streamed down her face as she spoke. I thought about how I would love to be in her shoes. After a few questions and answers, the group was dismissed for the afternoon break.

A VOLLEY OF HOPE

During the break, a group of us decided to play a game of beach volleyball. As we all gathered for the match, it was obvious the pall cast over the immersionists by their symptoms of withdrawal was lifting. You could almost sense a sort of enlightenment spreading. Although feelings of withdrawal may have still been with us, most people were beginning to move past them. The participants had begun to understand that they had a say in their health statuses. I overheard comments on Gail's inspiring reveal, while others in the group discussed the idea of using food to reverse disease. By the time the match ended, we had lots of immersionists playing. I am sure we had more players on the court than the rules normally allow, but everyone was laughing and having so much fun that it didn't matter. I couldn't remember a time when I'd felt this hopeful. Being surrounded by the other immersionists strengthened that hope for me, but there was more to it.

After the game, as I made my way back to my hotel room, it hit me. While my body may have been going through withdrawal, I hadn't once thought about leaving the volleyball match to catch my breath or get off my feet. With my body weight being what it was, just standing for more than fifteen minutes usually required a time-out—a place to sit down. I had been moving on the court for almost an hour and hadn't considered taking a break at all. It was strange. Something was definitely happening.

Despite wanting to take a shower as soon as I got to my room, when I saw that Michael was not there, I decided to take advantage of the privacy and call Iris first. We talked about how even though none of my symptoms had gone, I still somehow felt better. Even my mindset seemed to be shifting. Iris and I chatted for a bit longer, and then she handed the phone to Nigel. "Dad, are you skinny yet?" he asked. I laughed and told him I was working on it. Nigel and I talked about what things had been like for me at immersion so far, and about what had been going on at his school and with our family pets. I told him I loved and missed him dearly, and then we said our good-byes.

After freshening up, I headed downstairs to have dinner. My headache was nowhere near as intense as it had been earlier in the day. I noticed my appetite had returned. Walking into the dining room was a totally different experience than it had been that morning. People were talking and laughing again. I grabbed a plate and got in the buffet line. After fixing my plate, I headed to my usual table. Michael and the gang were waiting for me, and we all chatted and chuckled as we each ate a full meal for the first time all day. Before we finished, someone asked, "Are we meeting on the patio again tonight?" Everyone quickly agreed that we would. Our nights on the patio were becoming something to which we all looked forward in joyful anticipation. In fact, other immersionists soon asked if they could take part in our little tradition. Our patio party was growing.

We decided to call it a night at around 11 PM. Most of the group made plans to meet at Wendie Pett's exercise class before breakfast the next morning. As Michael and I walked back to our hotel room, we talked about everything that had happened since the start of immersion. We were both really excited about what we had experienced so far. After going through my nightly bedtime ritual, I climbed into bed and let my mind wander as I considered all the possibilities immersion held in store for me.

$\mathcal{D}$r. Stoll's Story

Breakfast on Day Three is usually quiet and subdued, as people have begun to feel the effects of the exercise schedule and experience symptoms of withdrawal from those items not available to them at the retreat, including junk food, caffeine, and tobacco. At around 8:15 AM, my family and I sat down to eat. I was enjoying a lovely bowl of oatmeal with blackberries, blueberries, and strawberries, and a green smoothie to drink, when the program's nurse, Lana, stopped by to give me an update and talk about one of the immersionists, John, who had not been feeling very well. She told me he had developed nausea and diarrhea overnight, so he would not be attending any lectures today.

I set my breakfast aside and went up to John's room to see how he was doing. He looked pale and weak, but he was still able to muster up a warm hello and a smile. After evaluating his vital signs, I explained to John that more than likely this illness was a case of withdrawal, which can occur when unhealthy foods have been removed from a person's diet. John couldn't believe the powerful hold junk food had on his body. I told him his body's almost overnight response to his new diet was evidence enough.

I left him my phone number and some coconut water for hydration, and told him Lana and our immersion physician, Dr. McGee, would check in on him in a couple of hours.

I got back downstairs shortly before 9 AM and walked into the ballroom to begin my lecture. As I stepped onstage, I saw many of the immersionists in the crowd had their heads down on their tables. It was clear to me that they, too, were in the throes of withdrawal. As a teacher, I was aware this wasn't the best time to give a long scientific speech. The audience was noticeably irritable and struggling to stay awake, but I knew what I had to say would offer clarity and hope to the program's participants, so I began.

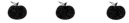

Good morning. Welcome to Day Three! By Day Three, people typically start to notice symptoms of withdrawal from junk food, which may include headaches, extreme fatigue to such an extent that you can't keep your eyes open (so, if you fall asleep during my lecture, I won't take it personally!), nausea, diarrhea, rashes, irritability, bad breath, a white tongue, aches and pains, intense cravings for comfort foods, and even vivid dreams. These symptoms emphasize the power unhealthy food has over you. It is eye-opening to recognize the agony your body experiences when it ceases to receive products full of sugar and salt that include a host of artificial and impossible-to-pronounce ingredients.

The good news is that once you get through the first three or four days of a new, healthy diet, your feelings of withdrawal should resolve. You will be free. Ironically, when you follow a plant-based diet, you may actually experience similar troublesome symptoms upon eating junk food again.

Would you like to know what is happening to your body right now as you transition to this better way of eating? It is an incredible story that is not widely known, but once you understand it, you will gain a new respect for and power over the food around you.

Let's begin by attempting to answer this question: Why do you eat? Have you ever stopped to ask yourself this simple question? The obvious answer is that your body needs calories, protein, fat, carbohydrates, vitamins, and minerals to survive and function. Beyond that basic understanding, however, why do you make certain food choices? Why do you sometimes feel the need to eat just before dinner or prior to going to bed?

A very revealing question to ask yourself as you pick up something to eat is: Why am I going to put this in my mouth? Sometimes the honest answer to this question is that you are putting the item in your mouth to satisfy your taste buds, not to supply any real nutritional requirements of your body. You aren't actually hungry.

True hunger directs you to consume foods that contain the raw materials needed for the countless biochemical reactions that occur in your body every second. Along with modifying signals from elsewhere in the brain, hunger is predominantly a signal from a part of the brain called the hypothalamus. It instructs you to seek out specific foods to meet your body's cellular needs. When you eat properly, your food provides energy to move your body, water to maintain hydration, fiber to feed the helpful bacteria in your digestive tract, and antioxidants to repair cell damage and promote healing.

Hunger signals may be disrupted by a number of external factors that cause you to confuse cravings for real hunger. These powerful false hunger signals can trigger you to eat unhealthy foods in larger quantities than you would ever plan on eating, and justify this behavior by convincing you that you were simply hungry. One key to your long-term success after this immersion will be to understand true and false hunger. You must learn to recognize when you are being motivated by cravings and not true physiological need.

The feeling of false hunger has a variety of possible causes, including thirst, habit, fatigue, boredom, stress, emotional pain, and depression. People frequently eat for the wrong reasons because they are responding to the wrong signals and don't know it. True hunger is simply your body's way of finding and consuming food that will meet its nutritional and caloric needs to maintain, heal, and animate itself throughout life. It is accompanied by particular biological signs, including a pulling sensation at the back of the throat, increased salivation, heightened sense of taste, and thoughts about specific foods that will meet your body's actual requirements—in other words, healthy foods.

Normal hunger is controlled by your body's hormones, receptors, and nerve input that detects the fat, protein, carbohydrates, and nutrients in your food. When the body needs calories and nutrients, several hormones that serve as hunger signals are released to the brain. Your stomach produces a hormone called ghrelin. This is the "hunger hormone" that rises when the stomach is empty, notifying the brain that you are hungry. At the same time, a lack of food in the gastrointestinal tract stimulates other hormones that signal hunger centers in the brain.

Your stomach contains neural stretch receptors that respond to the volume of food it contains. As you eat, your stomach fills up and expands, causing these receptors to stretch, which triggers a message that is sent to your brain. It takes about twenty minutes for this signal of fullness from your stomach to reach your brain, which then lets you know it's time to stop eating. This is why it is important to slow down and chew more. Research has shown that doubling the number of times you chew decreases the number of calories you consume by 12 percent (approximately twenty-four pounds of weight over one year) and increases your body's feeling of satiety, or fullness.[1,2]

When comparing the dietary stretch response brought about by 400 calories of oil—that's about three tablespoons—400 calories of chicken, and 400 calories of vegetables, the vegetables exert a significantly greater volume-based stretch, as well as earlier and greater satiety.

The Stomach's Stretch Response

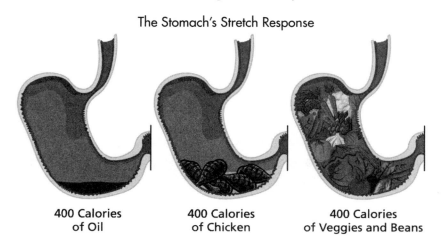

| 400 Calories of Oil | 400 Calories of Chicken | 400 Calories of Veggies and Beans |

In other words, plants provide a greater feeling of fullness at the same level of caloric intake as meat or processed food. This suggests that a plant-based diet will satisfy your hunger more quickly and keep you from snacking between meals.

Hunger officially ends, however, when the hormone leptin—the "satiety hormone"—rises after a meal in response to digestion. Leptin, which is essentially the opposite of ghrelin, tells your brain that your body's needs have been met, at which point your brain promotes a feeling of satisfaction.

Now, here is the important part: For some people, dieting has been shown to increase ghrelin and decrease leptin, causing more intense feelings of hunger and overwhelming urges to eat more food.[3] The best way to normalize these hormones, activate stretch receptors, and provide your body with an abundance of nutrients is to follow a plant-based diet of nutritious whole food. The volume and nutrient content of food in a plant-based diet will normalize the signaling pathway for hunger, leaving you with a feeling of fullness at the end of each meal.[4,5]

A plant-based diet also provides the joy of filling up your plate, which may prevent you from associating thoughts of restriction and scarcity—thoughts that drive hunger—with your daily diet. It allows you the freedom to eat food in abundance and variety. You won't have to count calories, or determine point values, or calculate percentages of macronutrients. It lets you enjoy your meal without effort and feel satisfied at its conclusion.

The human body requires over ninety nutrients to be healthy, including sixty minerals, sixteen vitamins, and numerous antioxidants. Deficiencies in these nutrients can stimulate hunger, but when unwholesome foods are consumed in response to hunger, your body continues to cry out for more nutrients to satisfy its cellular needs. Unfortunately, consumption of unhealthy food products does not meet the body's needs and tends to create false hunger or cravings for more of these types of food.

Foods chosen in response to your body's hunger pangs are frequently processed foods, candy, or fatty foods, which have few nutrients. These choices drive a cycle of undernourishment and overeating, causing chronic surges in leptin and insulin levels in the body. Frequent elevations in these hormones can lead to the cellular resistance previously mentioned, almost constant feelings of hunger, and inevitable weight gain.

THE POWER OF ADDICTION

Do you know what many experts consider the number one addiction in the United States? It is not drugs, alcohol, tobacco, sex, or gambling. It is processed food. The excessive amounts of sugar, fat, and salt in processed food stimulate the release of the neurotransmitter dopamine. Once this neurotransmitter binds to certain receptors, a sense of pleasure and reward is felt. Unfortunately, these receptors have also been associated with the brain's response to cocaine, methamphetamine, heroin, alcohol, tobacco, caffeine, gambling, videogames, political news, and sex.

We live at a time in history when the body's chemical reward system can be hyper-stimulated at any convenience store, checkout counter, or restaurant. Even at the electronics store or the office supply store, what do you pass on the way to the checkout? A gauntlet of chocolaty, sugary, fatty, and salty snacks. It is a challenge not to indulge your cravings. Repeated bite after bite of sugar, fat, and salt, however, causes more and more dopamine to be released, which leads to receptors becoming tolerant. After a while, larger quantities of these types of food will be required to bring about the same rewarding effects initially created by small amounts.[6] Greater amounts are required to stimulate the release of higher levels of dopamine to have any effect on intolerant receptors.

Further compounding this problem, researchers have discovered that dopamine receptors in the prefrontal cortex—the area of the brain responsible for organizing, planning, and choosing, as well as restraining impulsivity and compulsion—show less activity in obese subjects.[7] In other words, many people feel bad, eat large amounts of unhealthy food to feel better, know they shouldn't eat so much, feel it is beyond their powers to refuse, and then repeat this cycle, further saturating dopamine receptors and feeling worse than they had originally.

This cycle describes why moderation as a dietary recommendation does not work. In fact, it may perpetuate bad habits and increase risk of disease in some people. To put it simply: Would you recommend a moderate intake of cocaine to a cocaine addict?

We need to look at food addiction in the same way we view drug addiction. Remember that sugar, fat, and salt act on the same receptors that are stimulated by drugs. The only method of gaining control over addictive foods is a combination of abstinence, withdrawal, and support. A plant-based diet can help you in these pursuits, and the good news is that your receptors will begin to change and eventually return to normal once the excessive stimuli of sugar, fat, and salt are removed from your life.

To achieve freedom from food addiction, you must resensitize your reward system by abstaining from processed food, sugar, and fat for at least thirty days. During this time, it is important to change the way you think about these items. Ideas such as "can't," "off limits," "not allowed," "forbidden," and "cheat" actually set up your brain to crave them. Research has shown that when people are exposed to their favorite junk foods but not allowed to have them, they experience surges of dopamine in their brains, which incite intense cravings for these junk foods, making them extremely difficult to resist.[8,9]

I encourage a change in your thoughts on food, a change that will give you freedom and control. Instead of thinking of a certain food as forbidden, consider it allowable but not profitable to your health. You are in control because you may choose to eat any food at any time, but from now on you will make different choices. You possess the power to make wise decisions. Armed with your "why" and the knowledge of how hunger works biologically, you will choose to eat foods that support and enable your vision. You will gain new authority over food once your reward system has been renewed and is under control.

It is important to note that your biological reward system is normal and important. It is what helps you engage in new ventures, explore, learn, exercise, start a family, and pursue your dreams and passions. Throughout history, it has also served a vital role in finding food and creating memories of the locations of energy-rich foods. In fact, the dopamine reward system is connected directly to the emotional part of the brain known as the amygdala and the memory center of the brain known as the hippocampus. In other words, food has the ability to create emotional memories.

Have you ever tasted something that took you back to your childhood? Maybe it reminded you of your mother's pasta sauce simmering on the stove, or fresh cinnamon rolls coming out of the oven. Memories can be incredibly powerful. They can motivate you to eat certain foods that return you to a safe and happy place in your mind. We call them comfort foods for a good reason. They become a way to attain pleasure or find relief from pain, though you may not even realize it.

Now, which foods are typically chosen when stress and pain crop up in our lives? Broccoli, cauliflower, or kale? Not likely. Most of the time we choose ice cream, chips, chocolate, cheese, bread, or desserts, as these options quickly activate the reward center, and trigger positive emotional memories. They essentially act as pain and anxiety medications. The result of these choices is that we feel temporarily blissful and happy, and briefly escape our pain and stress. But these effects are short-lived. Ultimately, the source of stress and pain is not resolved, and guilt may appear, further compounding the problem.

In a recent study, rats that were addicted to cocaine were given the choice of continuing cocaine or switching to sugar. Remarkably, 94 percent of these rats chose sugar over cocaine. When the cocaine-addicted rats went into withdrawal, their symptoms were easily treated with sugar, confirming that both substances impact similar biochemical pathways.[10]

In another study, sugar and sweets created a more powerful neurobiological effect than intravenous (IV) heroin, suggesting that a double-chocolate cake with thick frosting may be the more powerful drug.[11] Similarly, a study at the University of Michigan gave chocolate-addicted subjects a drug called naloxone, which is used in emergency rooms to treat people that have overdosed on heroin, morphine, or other narcotics. These subjects were then placed in a room full of chocolate, cookies, and candy bars, and told they could eat as much as they wanted. Surprisingly, they did not desire the sweet treats and consumed very few of them.[12,13] The receptors that had been motivating their binge eating of chocolate were no longer controlling their appetites.

The high-sugar diet of today (on average, each person consumes one hundred and fifty pounds of sweeteners a year, including twenty-two teaspoons of sugar daily) results in overstimulation of the dopamine reward system, which can override self-control. In fact, high-fat, high-sugar foods silence the body's caloric-intake signals and stimulate consumption even when calories are not needed.[14] You might feel intense cravings, misinterpret these cravings as true hunger, seek out unhealthy food to satisfy these cravings, feel better, and then think you were just hungry. Your body didn't need those extra calories, though, and slowly weight begins to accumulate. In frustration, you seek a crash diet to get back on track. The deprivation and sacrifice of the diet is successful and you lose weight, but you still don't understand the power of food, so you celebrate with a piece of your favorite dessert, cheese, or snack.

Believing that your willpower is stronger than the draw of food, you begin to purchase unhealthy items again but make a commitment to eat them rarely. Like the siren's song, this food calls to you from the pantry, freezer, or refrigerator. You compromise with your desire and eat a little more of the junk food, still thinking you are in control. Your weight begins to rise and you begin to feel guilty, ashamed, and embittered. You condemn yourself for not having enough self-control to stick to your diet. Emotionally defeated, you don't feel good and seek to feel better by treating your pain and hopelessness with a couple of scoops of ice cream, a bar of chocolate, or a salty snack. You soon find yourself right back in the pleasure trap with no means of escape.

This day, however, I want you to feel encouraged by this fact: The door is always open. You can escape this trap at any time and leave this endless cycle behind. You can step into a new, joyful future unhindered by food addiction. Once you understand what is really happening, you can take back control of your health and change for good.

MORE THAN SUGAR

Although it is one of the main sources of food addiction, sugar is not the only culprit in the hijacking of your reward system. Many people I work with tell me, "I can give up sugar, but don't touch my cheese." Giving up cheese is often the last and strongest battle in the war against unhealthy food. But why is cheese so difficult to give up?

Let's put milk and cheese in context and first discuss the purpose and composition of dairy products. Milk is designed to provide all of the nourishment required by growing mammals, and each species has a unique milk composition. Monkey milk is different from water buffalo milk, which is different from cow milk, which is different from human milk. Cow milk is designed to grow a baby calf into a full-size cow in twelve to fifteen months and contains all the necessary ingredients for rapid growth, including higher levels of a protein called casein. Human milk is designed for slower body growth and more rapid neurologic development, and thus contains lower levels of casein, a distinctive amino-acid profile, higher lactose levels, and higher fat content than cow milk.

All milk contains morphine-like substances called casomorphins. (Remember that morphine is a painkiller used commonly in hospitals after surgery to dull pain.) These casomorphins are activated when gut bacteria break down casein into smaller protein chains.[15] They help calm nursing infants, improve the maternal-infant bond, slow down the gastrointestinal tract to prevent diarrhea, and motivate frequent feedings.

So, how does all this impact your choice to eat or not eat that extra slice of sharp cheddar? Milk contains approximately six grams of casein in an eight-ounce glass, and it takes ten pounds of milk to produce one pound of cheese. The casomorphin content of cheese is therefore many times greater than that of a glass of milk, and this difference is one of the reasons cheese but not milk frequently causes constipation. High levels of casomorphins combined with fat and salt can also cause cheese lovers to experience withdrawal symptoms due to a lack of cheese, including headaches, irritability, intense cravings, and fatigue. Subtle reinforcement of the desire for cheese occurs when that piece of Swiss suddenly makes the world feel right again—this association of cheese with good feelings becomes wired in your brain.

A CHANGE OF EMOTIONAL CLOTHING

In his book *The End of Overeating,* author Dr. David A. Kessler, former director of the Food and Drug Administration (FDA), shares a surprising secret as he states, "Food manufacturers have long been using focus groups to test for cravings and then designing their product for 'irresistibility' and 'crave-ability.' When a food scientist at Frito-Lay analyzed what determined 'irresistibility' five key influences were pinpointed: calories, flavor hits, ease of eating, meltdown and early hit. Companies know this and use this."

The industry knows that sugar, fat, and salt create emotional and biochemical reactions that bond you to a food. It also knows that when you don't eat that food, you experience withdrawal. Food products are crafted to create quick, intense, emotional hits that leave you craving more. You exchange your hard-earned money for brief moments of happiness, not realizing you have become enslaved to these food products. Millions of people are unwittingly dependent on junk food, and our culture enables this dependence by supporting an industry that exploits human biological pre-dispositions to sugar, fat, and salt.

Of course, chronic stress adds more kindling to the fire of food addiction. When you are under emotional stress, you are likely to grab a candy bar over a stalk of celery. The reason the sweet treat soothes your pain is found in your brain neurochemistry, as you now understand. Sugar, fat, and salt stimulate receptors in the brain—the same receptors stimulated by anti-anxiety med-ications and pain-relieving narcotics. As that first bite of junk food enters your mouth, your taste buds begin producing positive feedback.[16] For a brief time, your pain and anxiety are gone. You feel better, more hopeful, and in control. The dilemma, however, is that the root underlying your emotional stress has not been addressed, so the overeating loop continues.

The only way to overcome emotional eating is to get to the root of the problem. It sounds like a simple solution, but it can be challenging. I have worked with people whose history of abuse caused them to fear becoming attractive when they lost weight. Excess weight was protective to them, and as the pounds came off, they felt vulnerable, exposed, and fearful, and even-tually sabotaged any progress they had made to return to a safe place. Only once their deeper issues had been healed were they able to lose weight suc-cessfully and maintain a healthy lifestyle.

The first step in dealing with the root of your emotional issues is to change your emotional clothing, so to speak. Every day you get up and dress for the day, both physically and emotionally. Although you may not know it, sometimes you end up wearing the same emotional clothing for decades. And just as you can change your physical clothing, so, too, can you remove your old and tattered emotional garments.

For example, a man was traveling home on the subway after a frustrating and busy day at the office. He was tired and wanted some peace and quiet during the ride. At the next stop, a woman and her five-year-old son entered his car and sat right next to him. "Why me?" he muttered under his breath. Within minutes, the boy was bumping him, running up and down the aisle, and disobeying his mother's requests of him to sit down.

Anger began to well up inside the businessman and his patience came to an end when the boy stepped on his foot. Unable to contain himself, he yelled out, "Why can't you contain your son?" After an uncomfortable pause, the woman looked at him with tears in her eyes and said, "I am so sorry. We are just traveling home from his father's funeral and I guess he just doesn't know how to process what has happened."

Immediately, the man's anger disappeared and was replaced by compassion and patience. He experienced an instantaneous change in his emotional state by deciding to adjust his perspective. How many of you would have felt the same emotional transition in the face of such an honest exchange?

Today you can change your emotional clothing and remove some of those old, worn emotional garments that are doing you more harm than good. The chronic stress resulting from such emotions causes harmful physiological responses in your body. It affects thyroid function, bone density, muscle bulk, mood, immune function, and concentration. It also increases blood sugar, blood pressure, inflammation, abdominal fat, and appetite.[17] In fact, extensive research has documented the connection between your emotions and your immune system. Chronic stress disrupts your immune system, which may lead to impaired healing, susceptibility to infection, and elevated levels of inflammation, all of which can raise your risk of chronic disease.[18]

It is time to remove your fear, shame, guilt, anger, bitterness, and resentment. Eliminate pride and self-righteousness from your life, which only separate you from others. Choose forgiveness, kindness, gratitude, generosity, humility, love, peace, patience, and gentleness. Once you make the decision to do so, it takes only seconds to change your emotional clothing. I believe you will find your new outfit fits and feels a lot better than the old one. I can't wait to see it.

Before we take a break, I would like to leave you with an affirmation.

Today I choose to be free. Free from food addiction, free from emotional eating, free from unhealthy eating patterns.

I have the power of choice and the keys to be successful, and I will overcome. I will persevere, I will press on, and I will succeed.

Today I choose forgiveness. I forgive myself for everything I have done knowingly and unknowingly, and I give myself grace and patience to grow.

I choose to forgive all those in my life who have knowingly or unknowingly hurt me, and I release them and send them grace and blessings.

I choose to change my emotional clothing today. I will wear love, forgiveness, kindness, patience, gratitude, humility, kindness, and grace.

Thank you all for sharing this time with me today. Before you head off to enjoy the rest of Day Three, I would like to introduce you to our first reveal, who has kindly agreed to say a few words.

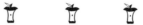

Right on cue, upbeat music began to fill the room at the conclusion of the lecture, lifting the spirits of the immersionists, who were fighting so hard to make it through such a difficult day. Gail walked onstage, nervous but excited to tell her story to the group. I knew her progress since leaving her last immersion would inspire her fellow team members. In fact, her store team leader had already let me know that Gail's new lifestyle had sparked in many workers and customers at that location a new attitude toward their own states of health.

Gail began by revealing the fact that she had lost over thirty pounds since leaving immersion, or four dress sizes. She explained how scared she had been to return home to her hectic schedule after being completely surrounded by healthy ideas at the retreat. It was plain to see, however, that she had decided to put her health first despite any struggles that might have reappeared in her day-to-day life. She had lost a significant amount of weight, stopped all her medications, gained a greater sense of what is and what is not healthy, and become a highly motivated individual. She concluded her speech by saying that she looked upon her new lifestyle as a means of enjoying many more happy years with her grandchildren. I could tell this last admission had made a powerful impact on the listeners.

After Gail's big reveal, I headed back to the room to change and spend some precious time at the beach with my family for some sun, sand, and surf. I make a point to factor in time spent on the beach during retreats because I believe the location is one of the best places to process the deeper issues of life.

While I sat on the beach with my family, I saw a woman from the immersion group walking toward us with tears streaming down her face. She stopped in front of the sand castle my kids and I had started to build and exclaimed, "I can't believe it!" I could see in her smile that she had good news to report. She went on to say, "I haven't been able to walk on the beach for twenty years because of the pain in my knees, and now, just three days into the program, I'm walking on the beach pain-free!"

She bent down to give me a hug and then continued down the beach, laughing with each step in the sand.

DAY FOUR

Milan's Story

On Day Four of immersion, I woke up at 5:45 AM, fifteen minutes before my alarm clock was scheduled to go off. As soon as I opened my eyes, I could tell something was different. For starters, my raging headache was noticeably absent. In addition, I was awake and alert, although I hadn't had a drop of caffeine in days. My mind was sharp and my thoughts were clear. I felt amazing. I didn't even think that was possible anymore without the help of caffeine.

I used the extra time to enjoy the quiet and feel grateful for the new day. Soon the alarm sounded, followed by our daily wake-up call. Michael got up and noticed I was already heading into the shower. He assumed I had experienced trouble sleeping the night before and had simply decided to get out of bed early. When I told him I had slept like a baby, he laughed. I told him I felt better than I had in years. Michael said he was feeling a lot better as well. I looked at him and said, "Maybe it was something we ate—or didn't eat." I told him I was going to go to the hotel gym and walk on the treadmill for twenty minutes before the morning exercise class. He asked if he could join me. "Absolutely," I said, "I would love the company."

After a quick shower, I decided to call Iris. She was still practically asleep when she answered the phone and asked me how I was feeling. I told her how alive I felt and how I'd even managed to wake up fifteen minutes early. She jokingly asked me if I had found a cup of coffee somewhere. I let her know that not only had I not had coffee, but also that I had never felt this good as a habitual coffee drinker. I also told her of my plan to walk on the treadmill before my morning exercise class. She laughed and said she was happy to hear I was feeling better. She then inquired about my agenda for the day. I let her know I would be attending a full morning of lectures, a cooking demonstration in the afternoon, and then a talent show after dinner. I told her I was going to write a poem about my immersion experience so far and read it at the show.

The talent show at the retreat had a bit of a reputation. Apparently, it had proved to be a blast for past attendees. As Michael and I headed downstairs, I mentioned my plan to write a poem despite not actually being much of a poet. He said he wasn't planning on participating in the show that evening, but told me I definitely should.

Once we got to the gym, I settled in on one of the treadmills in front of a huge window. I turned on my iPad, plugged in my earbuds, and tuned in to my favorite classical music station. I spent the time listening to music and thinking about my poem. I realized I had only the day to write it, as the talent show was scheduled to take place after dinner. I wanted the poem to be as honest as possible, as well as entertaining. About fifteen minutes into my trek, the title came to me. I would name my poem "From a Keg to a Six-Pack."

My waist had measured well over fifty inches at the start of immersion, and my dream was to have six-pack abs one day, so I thought this title would be clever while also allowing me to express my true feelings about where I was and where I hoped to be. As I walked on the treadmill, I was so focused on my poem that I lost track of time. The next thing I knew, Michael was signaling me that we needed to head to our morning exercise class. We quickly grabbed our water bottles and exercise mats and exited the gym.

Michael and I arrived at the oceanfront lawn area where the yoga class was being held at exactly 7 AM. It was packed, so we had to search for a place to set up our mats. The instructor began to announce the start of the class, so we found our spots as quickly as we could.

During the class, my mind was focused on my poem. I kept thinking about what I wanted to say. I was determined to talk about my decision to come to immersion, but I also wanted to discuss topics such as the food at the retreat and maybe even the withdrawal stage I had just gone through. I realized the poem could go in a lot of different directions. The sky was the limit. Poet or not, I was really getting excited about writing "From a Keg to a Six-Pack."

Michael and I headed back up to our room to drop off our exercise mats after class. We cleaned ourselves up, changed our clothing, and before heading back downstairs to breakfast I grabbed my iPad, opened up the "Notes" application, and typed "From a Keg to a Six-Pack" across the top of a blank note. I paused for a moment as I watched the cursor blinking on the screen. After a few seconds, I shut off my tablet, placed it under my arm, and headed downstairs with Michael.

When we entered the banquet hall, both Michael and I noticed that the other immersionists looked different. They seemed lively in a way they had not before. People were laughing and smiling. It was clear the withdrawal phases had ended for all of us. Michael and I found our usual table, placed our things at our seats, and then got in line for breakfast. The food looked and smelled so good. As I reached for a plate, I felt a tap on my shoulder. It was one of my new friends, Alex. She asked me how I was feeling. "Amazing," I replied. We chatted as we made our way through the buffet line.

I decided to try the buckwheat pancakes and warm tropical quinoa, along with a fresh blueberry smoothie to drink. I also grabbed an assortment of fresh fruit, including two of my favorite fruits, honeydew melon and cantaloupe. Once we had each made our choices, Alex, Michael, and I headed to our table to enjoy them.

Within minutes, we were joined by the rest of our little gang. As we began to eat our breakfasts, I asked if anyone was planning on participating in the talent show. Much to my surprise, almost everyone was hoping to take part in some way. Apparently, many of my new friends had heard about the immersion talent show from acquaintances who had attended prior retreats. We all wanted to know about each others' upcoming performances and the talents that would be on display.

There were singers, dancers, and even a magician in our group. Alex asked me what I was planning on doing as my talent, so I told her I was going to write and recite an original poem. She smiled and said, "I can't wait to hear your poem. I am sure it will be awesome!" I laughed and said, "We shall see."

I quickly finished my meal and excused myself from the table. I headed over to the ballroom where our lectures were being held so I could spend a little time working on my poem before the first speech of the day. I entered the room, took a seat at the back, and pulled out my iPad. I felt compelled to write. Something inside me was pushing me to do it. Except for Tom and a few other immersion staff members, I was the only one in the room. I put my earbuds in my ears and began clicking away on my iPad's keyboard. I looked up about fifteen minutes later to find the place full. Our first lecture of the day was about to begin.

NO FLUKE

Each lecture of Day Four would deal in some way with the notion that many common health conditions are caused or made worse by the standard American diet of high-fat, high-sugar meals. The lectures would also discuss how nutritional decisions could have dramatic effects on many types of illness. In other words, while food can hurt us, it can also heal us.

Dr. Stoll began his first lecture by talking about the way in which crops are grown and the connection between soil health and food quality. He then went on to explain the troubling way in which modern diet fads focus too much on individual concepts such as calories, carbohydrates, protein, or fat, and neglect the importance of whole food in all its complexity.

On a break between lectures, I went out to the patio and noticed the immersion staff once again performing blood pressure tests. I quickly got in line to have my blood pressure taken. I wanted to see if my recent reading had been a fluke. When the time came to have my blood pressure taken, I sat down and pulled up my shirt sleeve. A few moments later I heard, "100 over 77." It was official. I was definitely not the same Milan that had arrived a mere four days earlier. I was changing from the inside out.

SIMPLE TRUTH

I returned to my seat after the break. The next round of information picked up where the previous speech had left off. Dr. Stoll provided us with a brief history of plant food, explaining how real, whole food contains numerous health-promoting substances working in combination, and suggesting that isolated nutrients could never equal the power of a food in its natural form. He talked about supplements and how the products made by this billion-dollar industry were usually unnecessary and often ineffective. He was adamant that if people simply followed a plant-based diet of whole food, they would receive more than enough essential vitamins and minerals. Furthermore, they would get these important nutrients in their ideal forms while also receiving any complementary substances that might enhance their overall effectiveness.

I sat in my seat thinking about how so much of the dietary advice we had been given as children was, at best, misguided. The fact that the ideas being shared at the retreat were not common knowledge seemed absolutely crazy to me. I realized I had a duty to seek out the truth instead of merely accepting what I had been raised to believe as true. Until I entered immersion, I had always assumed my health was not something I could control to any significant degree. I felt it was something I simply had to deal with and live through. Immersion was teaching me this was not the case.

Before I knew it, we were released for lunch. Michael and I joined our gang in the banquet hall and discussed the upcoming talent show. The grand prize winner of the show would win a brand new Vitamix blender, so I knew competition would be fierce. I realized I would need to find more time to work on my poem if I was going to have it ready for the competition. I told Michael and the rest of the group that I'd better use the lunch break to get some writing done. Excusing myself from the table, I grabbed my plate and made my way to the patio. I settled into a chair facing the ocean and pulled out my iPad. Ideas for my poem began to flow from my mind to my fingertips. Words were coming to me so fast that my fingers could barely keep up to type them. I was in the zone. In what seemed like the blink of an eye, lunchtime was over, and I headed back to the ballroom to meet Michael and attend a cooking class we had both been anticipating greatly.

FULL-FLAVORED HEALTH

In addition to exercise classes and eye-opening lectures, the retreat also offered a couple of cooking demonstrations run by world-renowned vegan chef Chad Sarno. I was thrilled to be attending one of the retreat's cooking demonstrations because I had heard chef Sarno would be teaching us how to take our new plant-based diet to an even higher level in our own kitchens. This was a crucial aspect of the program, in my opinion. If I couldn't figure out how to cook truly delicious and flavorful plant-based meals, I knew I would not be able to sustain this lifestyle.

Within minutes of chef Sarno beginning the class, the entire room was filled with the scent of onions and garlic sautéing. He was cooking up a veggie stew, and making it all look really simple. One of Dr. Stoll's daughters passed around samples of chef Sarno's tasty creation once it was ready, and it dawned on me that not only would I be able to go home and cook great-tasting plant-based dishes, but I would also be able to make cooking an activity for my whole family. I was so excited to start.

Chef Sarno ended his cooking class by explaining how important it was for us to have fun with the meals we would make at home. He let us know that eating healthy did not mean eating bland or boring food. He reminded us that a nutritious meal could also be fun and full of flavor.

As chef Sarno finished his demonstration and began cleaning up his work area, Dr. Stoll took the stage and introduced the second and final reveal of the retreat. I noticed Alex stand and begin to make her way toward the stage. I just couldn't believe it. Alex had been hanging out with us at our nightly patio parties since I had arrived at immersion. Prior to her reveal, I had actually thought Alex might be part of the immersion staff in some way, as I had noticed her helping out on the day we had all gotten blood work done. I had simply never bothered to ask her about it.

I glanced over at Michael, who looked equally surprised, and we sat in silence as Alex shared her story. As she spoke, a picture taken of her before immersion appeared on a screen behind her. You could hear gasps throughout the room. Alex was about five feet tall, maybe even a bit shorter. She told us she had lost over thirty pounds since her last immersion. Because of her small stature, the weight loss made her look like a completely different person. Her "before" picture didn't look anything like her. The bags under her eyes were now gone and the swelling in her face had disappeared. She actually appeared as though she had never been overweight. She had gone from a size twelve to a size two. She wasn't merely thinner, she was stunning. Alex had not just lost weight; she had completely transformed herself.

Alex described how her new lifestyle was affecting every aspect of her life in a positive way. She talked about how eating healthy was benefiting her two small children as well as her mother, who was obese and suffering from an array of chronic diseases. Alex was happy to tell us that her mother was now starting to find some relief from these health conditions since switching to a plant-based diet of whole food. After a brief question-and-answer session, the reveal concluded and we were given a long break before dinner.

During this free time, I happened to see Alex standing on the beach. I approached her and congratulated her on her amazing transformation. I asked her what the toughest part of the entire process had been for her. She replied, "Understanding that my journey was my journey." I asked her what she meant by that and she explained that after immersion many people close to her had tried to talk her out of sticking with her new lifestyle. It had seemed as though her friends and family were, perhaps unintentionally, trying to derail her efforts. She then told me it had also been difficult to learn how to love herself again. Both of her statements surprised me, but they made sense.

Alex and I walked back to the hotel and, before we parted, she said, "Milan, this immersion experience will be what you make of it. This is your moment, so embrace it!" I smiled and thanked her for her time. Then I headed up to my room to put the finishing touches on my poem.

My talk with Alex had given me clarity. Alone in my room, I sat down at the desk and poured everything I had into my poem. Line after line, it all began coming together. Within an hour, I was done. "From a Keg to a Six-Pack" was complete. I sat there for a moment, reading through what I had written.

THE TALENT SHOW

After putting the finishing touches on my poem, I jumped in the shower to freshen up before dinner. I knew I would need to head straight to the talent show after eating, so I wanted to make sure I was ready. Before heading back downstairs, I took a moment to call Iris and Nigel. Nigel actually answered the phone. "Hey, Daddy!" he said excitedly. Nigel and I talked for about five minutes. He filled me in on everything that had been going on in his life, and I told him how great I felt now that my feelings of withdrawal had passed. I told Nigel I loved him, and then he handed the phone over to his mom.

"How is the poem coming along?" she asked. I told her I had completed the poem and would be sure to have someone film my performance so she could see it. Then I told her about Alex's reveal. I have no doubt Iris could hear the enthusiasm in my voice as I shared with her all the details of Alex's transformation. At the end of our conversation, Iris and Nigel both wished me luck at the talent show before I hung up and read through my poem one last time before going to dinner.

The banquet hall was abuzz with talk of the big event that would follow that evening's meal. I saw people practicing their acts, while others were going over the details of their upcoming performances. It was obvious everyone was excited. I quickly made a plate of food and headed over to my favorite table, where the whole gang was already waiting.

As I took my seat, Michael asked me if I had been able to finish my poem. I smiled and said I had. He then asked me if I was nervous. "Strangely enough, I'm not," I said. After dinner, our entire group made its collective way to the ballroom, where the talent show would be held.

A DJ was setting up in the upper right-hand corner of the room. In the middle of the space were rows of chairs for the audience. The judges' table stood opposite the DJ's turntables on the other side of the room. Since it was actually Halloween night, there was a huge box of props between the DJ set-up and the judges' table. My group found seats in the front row, and then Tom took the stage to announce the rules of the event. There would be three judges, two of which would be the immersion reveals. The final judge would be Tom's wife, Andrea. Tom let the room know that whoever wanted to perform would need to sign up at the DJ's table.

After signing up for a slot, I realized I would be the final act to perform. I took my seat alongside the rest of my friends and the show began. The first few acts were fun and silly. Next came a few people who displayed fantastic singing talent. Jesse was a female singer who had the most incredible voice. She stepped to the microphone and sang a song by Adele. From the moment she opened her mouth, the entire room gasped in astonishment. Her voice cut through the room like a warm knife through butter. Her performance was breathtaking. She scored twenty-nine points out of a possible thirty. I realized the only way I could win was to get a perfect score.

We reached the end of the show and Tom took the stage to introduce me. My stomach was in knots. I heard him say, "Please welcome our very own 'Big Sexy' to the stage!" I grabbed my iPad and walked up to the microphone. I told everyone I wanted to share an original poem about my immersion experience. I cleared my throat and began to read.

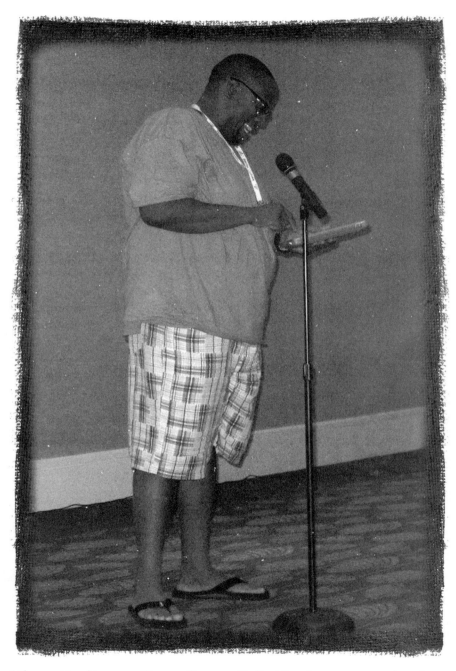

Milan reciting his poem "From a Keg to a Six-Pack" at the immersion talent show.

From a Keg to a Six-Pack

Once upon a time . . . . Well, back when I was thin
I did lots of cool stuff like shoot hoops and swim
I could eat whatever I wanted and never gain a pound
Stay up late and drink a couple of beers . . . . Awwww, it was going down
That is until one day about fifteen years ago I started to put on a little bit
    of weight
It hit my thighs, then my butt, my gut and my face
At first it was cool because back then I was a bean pole
Six foot four about a buck eighty is what I weighed. . . .
    Super Sexy from head to toe
Hey ladies, I am just saying. . . .
Anyway, the weight kept coming pound after pound
After a while I went from super sexy to just plain old round!
After a few more years I guess it could be said
I had officially gone from a six-pack to a keg
Now, I know kegs are fun at parties and whatnot
But they ain't real cool when you have trouble even putting on socks
See my feet back then . . . . Child, please
Every day that went by my belly got closer to my knees
Anyway, later in life I took a new job
At a place I used to make fun of
Because everyone there I thought of as food snobs
But this place, WFM, is like no other
They actually cared about my well being instead of just my production
WFM wanted to see me be the best me I could be
So they put me on a plane and flew me out by the sea
Coming from Colorado, where right now it's cold
I thought, hmmm . . . . What the hell. . . . I'll go hang out with Dr. Stoll
It's a week of fun in the sun; I can work on my tan
Hit the beach, listen to a of couple lectures; I'll be cool like a fan
Right out the gate, Dr. Sean makes me cry
Then Dr. Stoll and Dr. Klaper tell me how the food I am eating is going
    to make me die

Now I am thinking, Florida, hmmm . . . not so cool
Don't even get me started on all the salad and all the poop
I came here thinking that this was fat camp
But knowledge is power, so now I am leaving here a champ
Listen, if you guys don't remember anything I just said,
    please retain this one fact
After I leave here I am putting in the work
And the next time y'all see me I will have gone from a keg to a six-pack!

The crowd hung on every word of my poem as I read it. They laughed out loud as I talked about what immersion had been like for me so far. When I spoke about my plans and dreams for the future, I felt the crowd acknowledge my readiness to shed my "Big Sexy" persona.

I finished reading and the room burst into applause. People screamed and yelled as they all stood on their feet and clapped. Now it was up to the judges. After about ten minutes or so, the verdict was in. Judge number one gave me a perfect ten. Judge number two gave me a perfect ten. Judge number three would make the final call. I got an eight.

I lost the talent show by a hair. The funny thing was that even though I had lost the big prize, I knew I had won something much greater. I hugged Jesse and congratulated her on her victory. I knew I had accomplished more than I had ever thought possible just by coming to immersion. For me, in that moment, it was enough.

After the performances, the DJ began to play music and the crowd began to dance. We all laughed and moved like never before. It felt as though we were all celebrating a rebirth. The party went on for at least another two hours, and afterwards our little group met on the patio. Everyone told me how moved they had been by my poem.

We chatted for several hours, and by midnight we decided to pack it in. Michael and I went up to our room and got ready for bed. We lay there talking about the unbelievable experience immersion was proving to be. Michael told me he thought I should have won the talent show. I let him know I had won. With that, we turned off the light and went to sleep.

$\mathcal{D}$r. Stoll's Story

My wife slipped out of the room early in the morning for a walk on the beach and an exercise class. I had encouraged her to take some time for herself during immersion because she had certainly earned it, always taking incredible care of our family, six children and all. Her absence meant I was in charge of getting the children up and ready for the day. My multitasking skills were put to the test as I made sure baths, clothes, hair, teeth, room cleanup, and even bathroom duties were taken care of before breakfast at 8 AM.

As I entered the banquet hall with my family, I noticed the atmosphere in the room had completely changed. I saw more smiles and energy than I had seen the day before. It was clear the withdrawal symptoms that had been plaguing the immersionists had started to fade. The participants were beginning to experience some of the many benefits a nutritious plant-based diet has to offer. Several people came over to me during breakfast to tell me how overjoyed they were, enthusiastically saying that their diabetes or blood pressure medications were being reduced or discontinued by the in-house physician after only three days of following this new lifestyle. Their genuine and heartfelt smiles and embraces were the best reward I could imagine.

The group was now more alert and engaged. They were hopeful about immersion, the power of food, and their own futures. By 9 AM, everyone had taken a seat in the ballroom for the morning lecture and I began my talk by asking an important question.

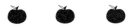

Why are we spending an entire week talking about food? It is because, according to the United States Department of Agriculture, the average

American consumes almost two thousand pounds—nearly a ton—of food each year. Nearly 63 percent of that amount is made up of processed food; 25 percent is made up of animal products; and 12 percent is made up of vegetables and fruits. This story gets more alarming when you see that the vegetable and fruit percentage consists mostly of potatoes—mainly in the form of french fries—ketchup, and fruit juice.

So, what are your yearly pounds going to consist of? That's the single most important health-related question of your life. No other decision will have the same effect on your health as the food you choose to eat three times a day, every day, over the course of eighty or more years. Please consider for a moment the positive or negative impact those pounds of food can have on your health over a lifetime. This choice can affect your health, finances, relationships, spiritual life, work, and future opportunities. Yet most people spend more time researching their next smart phone than they do food that can create optimal health. To top it all off, the diet industry and the media in general often put forth conflicting information, leading to a sense of confusion and mental fatigue when it comes to making healthy food choices.

Every day, millions of people exchange their hard-earned money for food that tantalizes their taste buds for a few seconds, fills their bellies for a couple of hours, but causes them to feel unfulfilled. Over time, their bodies become starved for nutrients and slowly grow susceptible to degenerative lifestyle-related diseases, including heart disease and type 2 diabetes.

I would like to begin to write a new story of food with you, one that will provide you with knowledge, inspiration, and renewed hope. These days, the wonder of food has been eliminated through industrialization, processing, packaging, marketing, and excessive focus on its components instead of its wholeness. The treasure that is real food has been lost, replaced by worthless novelties. It is time to remember that whole food is beautiful, potent, and delicious.

Before we write a new story of food and move forward, however, I want to dispel a few old concepts that may be holding you back. Over the last hundred years, public opinion has embraced the idea that food should be inexpensive. In 1950, the average person spent 34 percent of his or her income on food and worked almost fifteen days to pay for healthcare costs. In 2012, the average person spent 13 percent of his or her income on food and worked close to sixty days to pay for healthcare costs.[1] We are spending less money on food, but we are also unhealthier and paying more to try to heal ourselves.

Is it any coincidence that the cheapest food available is made of mostly sugar and processed grains?[2] Food should be one of the most important aspects of your monthly budget because it can provide you with the means to improve your health and, in turn, lower your healthcare expenses. This does not necessarily mean, however, that you'll need to break the bank in order to eat well. Don't use presumed cost as an excuse not to eat well. One Harvard study concluded, "Although spending more money was associated with a healthy diet, large improvements in diet may be achieved without increased spending. The purchase of plant-based foods may offer the best investment for dietary health."[3]

Although a plant-based diet of whole food may sound boring, it is anything but. In reality, the Western diet is the boring option—it offers only a handful of different flavors, with salt being its predominant spice. Healthy plant-based meals present numerous opportunities to introduce your taste buds to amazing flavors while their nutritious ingredients fulfill the biochemical needs of your cells.

Finally, when it comes to diet, the value attached to convenience has been sorely misplaced. People use drive-through windows at fast food restaurants because their lives are too busy, but then they plop down on their couches to watch hours of television! They don't realize the true price of convenience: More time spent in waiting rooms at doctors' offices and more income put toward managing diseases resulting from making convenient food choices rather than good ones. When you invest your time in a healthy diet, you actually end up keeping more money in your pocket and having more time on your hands, so don't be fooled by the drive-through window.

FOR THE LOVE OF THE SOIL

The story of real food begins when a seed is placed in soil. Water absorbed by the seed activates chemical reactions that cause it to germinate, or sprout. Once the seed has germinated, an amazing relationship develops between the living soil and the growing plant.

Soil is not just dirt that stains your carpet or children's clothing. It is composed of silt and clay, and infused with leaves, sticks, hair, and other organic material that might fall to the ground. Earthworms burrow through soil, eating organic materials and then leaving behind open channels for water, air, and roots to access, as well as waste products, which add minerals and nutrients back to the soil, maintaining healthy soil.

Soil is full of good bacteria and fungi that support the health of the plants growing in it. For instance, microrrhizal fungi found in rich soil actually pierce the root hairs of a plant, growing into and becoming part of that plant's root system. The fungi receive nutrients and sugar in exchange for the minerals and water it gathers from the soil and gives to the plant.[4,5] In this way, the plant becomes able to extend its reach for valuable water and minerals. Both the plant and fungi flourish because of their symbiotic relationship.

When soil is rich in minerals and living organisms, it produces a robust plant that can actually become resistant to pests and disease. Healthy plants don't require pesticides and herbicides to grow; they are able to fight disease through their own natural mechanisms, including the production of compounds called phytochemicals.

When grown in good soil, produce such as strawberries, blackberries, kale, and broccoli end up containing minerals, vitamins, and abundant phytochemicals, which can help the human body grow, fight infection, repair DNA damage, reduce inflammation, regulate hormones, and even kill cancer cells. When you eat a plant or its fruit, your body absorbs its minerals, vitamins, and phytochemicals, which work in much the same way they do in the plant or fruit, optimizing cellular health. All you have to do is enjoy a wonderful meal of plant-based food, finish with a bowl of your favorite berries, and voilà! Hundreds of phytochemicals, minerals, and vitamins go to work strengthening, repairing, and healing your body.

Organic farmers love soil. They can spend hours talking about it because they understand that the health of their soil directly correlates to the health of the people consuming the food grown in it, as well as to the health of the ecosystem. Industrialized agriculture doesn't focus on soil health but rather on crop yield. This approach leads to short-sighted farming that repeatedly tills topsoil and applies pesticides and herbicides that damage the soil's living organisms, including earthworms. This damage weakens plants and makes them unable to defend themselves without pesticides, fungicides, or herbicides. These chemicals are then added to industrial crops to protect plants and increase yield. This troublesome cycle inevitably results in depleted soil.

Numerous articles suggest that this misplaced emphasis on crop yields and not soil health, which began in the 1940s, has resulted in produce with a lower nutrient content.[6] A recent study comparing the mineral composition of twenty fruits and vegetables found significant declines in all minerals except phosphorus—a common element in modern fertilizer.[7] In 1958, one apple contained 4.8 mg of iron. Today, you would need to consume twenty-six apples to obtain the same amount of iron. Organic produce consistently contains higher levels of phytochemicals and antioxidants, and a comprehensive review of available studies on the subject found organic produce to offer 25 percent more nutrients across the board when compared with conventional produce. These additional nutrients, coupled with lower lifetime exposures to pesticides and herbicides, make clear the cumulative benefit of organic fruit and vegetables.

If you find the cost of organic food too high, however, adding more conventional produce to your diet will still yield significant health benefits. Plant-based food grown in healthy soil possesses abundant vitamins and minerals, but even conventional options offer a large amount of nutrients.

The health benefits and disease-preventing power of whole plant-based food is clear and irrefutable.[8,9,10] For instance, chlorophyll, the chemical that gives plants such as kale and spinach their green color, acts as an anti-inflammatory agent in the human body.[11,12] It is interesting to note that the chemical structure of chlorophyll is nearly identical to that of hemoglobin, a molecule in red blood cells that carries oxygen from the lungs to the rest of the body. This similarity may explain why several studies have shown wheatgrass to improve blood markers in children afflicted with a blood disorder known as thalassemia major, resulting in fewer blood transfusions being required by patients.[13,14]

It is also important to note that it is the combination of minerals, vitamins, phytochemicals, plant fiber, and other healthy elements that exerts positive effects on the body. When it comes to consuming plant food, the whole is greater than the sum of its parts, so try not to focus on a single or isolated nutrient in regard to the benefits of eating produce. When you eat a plant whole, each bite is like swallowing a nutritional symphony, as each instrumental component plays its part perfectly and harmoniously in your body. This symphonic effect is multiplied when more plant-based options are added to your plate, creating a complex mixture of micronutrients that synergistically begin to work together throughout your entire body within an hour after you finish your meal.[15,16]

NOT ALL CALORIES ARE CREATED EQUAL

Not all calories are created equal in their nutrient contents or physiological effects, as made clear by research or any comparison of a Twinkie with broccoli. Of course, the calories in broccoli are far superior to the same number of calories in a Twinkie, but let's take a look at the difference just for fun.

One cup of broccoli contains 54 calories, 3.7 g of protein, and 5 g of fiber. It also has over thirty vitamins and minerals, seven phytochemicals, and a good dose of chlorophyll, all of which boost the immune system. Compare these numbers with one-third of a Twinkie cake, which has 45 calories, thirty-seven ingredients (including 8 g of sugar, 2 g of fat), no fiber, and almost no protein. These qualities leave you feeling empty and craving more. When it comes to food, always remember that every bite can either harm or heal you.

A calorie is simply a measurement that tells you how much energy is in a food. It may be defined as the amount of energy needed to raise 1 g of water by 1°C, referring to the measurement of temperature known as Celsius. It was first defined by French scientists in 1825, and then used by W.O. Atwater in 1887 to describe food and food composition within academic circles. It first captured the public's attention, however, during World War I, when the FDA used the calorie as a tool to promote rationing of wheat, sugar, and meat. At that time, some restaurants even featured calorie counts on their menus, along with statements and slogans promoting miserly eating and calorie-counting patriotism.

Then, in 1918, Dr. Lulu Hunt Peters, a physician who personally struggled with her own weight, wrote the first modern diet book, entitled *Diet and Health,* which went on to become a bestseller for the next five years. In the book, Dr. Peters promoted calorie counting and calorie restriction as the most scientific and reliable methods of maintaining a healthy body weight. The calorie has become a mainstay in the majority of diet books that have come out since. With a calculator in hand at mealtimes, anyone could achieve the "perfect" body weight.

To prove the connection between calorie counting and weight management, one researcher lost twenty-seven pounds in ten weeks on a diet that featured Oreos, Twinkies, and other junk food. He validated the point that counting calories leads to weight loss, but he was no healthier at the end of his diet.[17] Unfortunately, appearance is frequently the reason behind counting calories, leading to unhealthy dietary strategies that fuel frustration, guilt, and hopelessness. Today, the calorie stands supreme in a diet industry that has people counting, sweating, burning, starving, and working off those pesky little units of energy.

So, what is the biggest problem with this calorie-based concept? It reduces food down to a simple mathematical formula and ignores the breathtaking complexity of food and its profound impact on every cell in your body. It also overlooks the psychological reality that none of us can count calories year after year without becoming so frustrated that we dump our calculators in the trash and add another scoop of ice cream to our bowls in rebellion. Additionally, the majority of people underestimate the number of calories they eat and overestimate the calories they burn off. This leaves them hopelessly chasing that elusive caloric balance.[18,19] The fact is that calories do not always equal health. It is the nutritional content of your food that ultimately determines your well-being. Nevertheless, nutrient-rich plant-based food can optimize both your caloric intake and your health.

Researchers have confirmed the benefits of a plant-based diet in maintaining optimal weight, along with high meal satisfaction. In terms of the energy density of food, which may be defined as the number of calories contained per gram, they found that the low energy density of a plant-based meal, along with its high fiber and low calorie counts, provided the same level of meal satisfaction as a high-energy meal that included food choices common to the standard American diet.[20]

People can essentially eat more food, feel fuller, and enjoy their meals, despite eating fewer calories.[21] The restaurant industry has understood for a long time that a large plate and a feeling of fullness at the end of a meal influence the perceived satisfaction of that meal.[22] A plant-based diet of whole food provides you with an opportunity to pile your plate high and even go for a second helping without necessarily consuming too many unnecessary calories. The abundance of food both visually and perceptively produces a sense of freedom that can catalyze long-term change.

THE POWER OF WHOLE FOOD

For most of human history, people have thought of food in terms of wholeness. A fig was a fig; wheat was wheat; a pomegranate was a pomegranate; and so forth. This simple mindset helped maintain clarity in regard to eating. I sincerely believe we are wired to think holistically about food, not in the reductionist way we are being convinced to think today, fixated on calories, carbs, fat, and protein. Our obsession with low-carb, low-fat, high-protein, low-calorie diets goes against human nature and injects confusion, bargaining, and food myths into our daily meal choices. It is more fun to create a dish in the kitchen around examples of whole food rather than design a recipe based on scientific research on individual nutrients.

For millennia, food was food. Then came the Age of Enlightenment, and science began to probe past the peel to find that the simplicity of food was a lot more complex than we had thought. By 1827, the English chemist William Prout had discovered that food could be divided into the macronutrients of protein, fats, carbohydrates, and water. Soon after that, the connection between minerals in soil and plants was made, and by 1912, the Polish biochemist Casimir Funk had coined the term "vitamines" to label the vitally important substances in plants, which were found to prevent diseases such as beriberi, a condition caused by vitamin B_1 deficiency. The public, amazed by the power of vitamins, believed these compounds had the power to impart good health beyond simply curing diseases of deficiency. Before long, vitamins began to be bottled and sold. A new industry was born.

Over the next thirty-five years, many more vitamins were discovered, and by the early 1980s, phytochemicals had been identified as the source of color, taste, odor, and protection in plants. Today, more than seven thousand have been discovered, and more will be discovered in the years to come.

What can we learn from the history of plant food? It teaches us that we don't have a complete understanding of plants, that there is always something new to be discovered. Handfuls of isolated nutrients will never equal the power of food in its whole form.[23] Scientific exploration may enhance our understanding of food, which is very exciting and worthwhile, but we must not forget the dietary foundation of so many healthy, long-lived cultures: whole plant food.

A diet of whole plant food affords you the unique opportunity to reconnect to abundance, creativity, and fulfillment when it comes to your meals. For a number of reasons, a plant-based lifestyle provides the greatest opportunity for success in terms of your health and well-being. The variety of flavors satisfy, the fiber content fills the stomach and creates a sense of fullness, the phytochemicals turn off hunger signals, a visibly full plate satisfies the eyes and mind, and there is no feeling of deprivation to alter hunger centers in the brain. When you focus on the whole and not the parts, you will have all you need.

YOUR TIPPING POINT

I would like to end this lecture with a concept that emphasizes the importance of making the best decisions you can make today. Most things in life don't just happen out of nowhere; there is usually a series of events that build over time until a tipping point is reached, and then change seems to occur abruptly.

My patients often ask me, "Doc, how did this happen?" They are stunned by a diagnosis of type 2 diabetes or dementia. They are shocked by a heart attack. They are baffled by severe arthritis of the hip. Many are bowled over by a diagnosis of illness and point to their last physical exams, which showed a clean bill of health. They don't realize their illnesses were growing subclinically—below the sensitivity of modern medical testing—and their "normal" test results emboldened the idea that they would escape any repercussions of their poor dietary and lifestyle choices. They don't realize they have reached their tipping points.

Health problems oftentimes reflect decades of decisions, compensations, and events that have slowly resulted in these conditions. Bite by bite, step by step, one stressful day after another, one drink or smoke after another, we neglect our bodies' cries for nutrients, exercise, and rest, and ignore our emotional burdens.

The body can endure repeated trauma for years. It has been constructed with incredible resiliency, and it will pull from its reserves as long as possible to meet demand. Eventually, though, once enough cells have been injured, dysfunction occurs, followed by disruption, and then disaster. Heart disease, type 2 diabetes, dementia, autoimmune disease, osteoarthritis, osteoporosis, and even cancer are a few of the most common diseases that generally have an incubation period of years to decades.

Take, for example, atherosclerotic heart disease, or hardening of the arteries. Arteries on the surface of the heart supply blood to this muscle so that it may continue its work of beating eighty times a minute, or forty-two million times a year. When they become clogged with calcified plaque, this plaque can inhibit and block the flow of blood. The muscle, still contracting, needs oxygen and nutrients provided by blood, but now it is not receiving blood effectively. The heart becomes starved of oxygen, which leads to a heart attack.

Autopsy studies have found evidence of early heart disease in children as young as six years old, who displayed early signs of atherosclerosis.[24] Another study showed that one of six teenagers had even more significant atherosclerotic problems.[25] A review of autopsies of trauma victims in their thirties revealed an approximate 77 percent rate of atherosclerosis.[26] Finally, it has been estimated that over 95 percent of men over the age of eighty who have lived the average American lifestyle have atherosclerosis.[27] This progression is not the result of aging, though, but rather of repeated damage to the body.

The tipping point of heart disease is a heart attack. The tipping point of type 2 diabetes is when your doctor says you have elevated blood sugar and writes a prescription for oral medication or insulin. It may take only a brief moment to discover your body is ailing, but it typically takes more than a moment to become unwell. It is often the culmination of years of unhealthy choices. Sometimes there are warnings that are ignored, of course, and you may reach the point at which changing your diet and lifestyle will not be able to reverse all the damage done over the years.

Another way to think of accumulated cellular injury and the tipping point of disease is to consider credit card debt. Have you ever been met with an unwelcome surprise upon opening your credit card statement? *How did this happen?* you might have wondered as you looked at the amount due. It was one fun swipe at a time—a purchase here and a purchase there—that led to that number. Did you ignore the bill, and, if so, were there consequences? The same scenario may apply to your body.

If you are facing disease, you need to reverse accumulated injury. In other words, you need to pay off your health debt and avoid building it back up again. To do so, you must change the unhealthy behaviors that led to that debt, and plant-based food, stress management, physical activity, and proper rest are valuable currencies.

The good news to think about as you go to bed tonight is this: Your health debt can be minimized and, in most cases, paid off completely in a relatively short period of time. As you begin to make the necessary adjustments to take your health out of the red and put it back in the black, remember the following affirmation.

I am grateful for plant food and its abundance of choices and tastes.

I am grateful for my body and the new hope I have that I can change and will change.

When I see whole plant food, I will pause to remember its story and give thanks for the gift of this delicious, nourishing food.

I believe I can overcome my health tipping point and reverse the trend through the power of choice that has been given to me.

I hope you all enjoy the cooking demonstration this afternoon, which promises to be full of surprises.

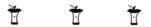

Later that day, after a wonderfully educational cooking class given by the very talented chef Chad Sarno, I introduced the second reveal of the week, Alex, to the immersionists. They were stunned to see Alex walk up to the microphone. She looked so healthy that many attendees had assumed she was part of the staff. Alex shared her inspiration for attending immersion the first time, which was a coworker who had returned from a retreat with renewed vitality, beautiful skin, and a positive perspective on life that was infectious.

She described herself as having been overweight, unhappy, lacking the energy required to care for her family properly, barely able to make it through the day, frightened by a strong family history of heart disease and diabetes, and secretly yearning to be a role model for her kids.

She said her life-changing moment came during her first immersion when she realized whole plant foods were beautiful and important to life, and that they could help her feel renewed. She also mentioned that seeing my children happily eating healthy meals had been a pivotal moment of the retreat. It had made her believe change was possible for her whole family. Since her initial immersion experience, she had lost approximately thirty pounds—a lot for someone who was only about five feet tall—taken inches off her waist, and improved her cholesterol readings. Moreover, she now woke up each day feeling rested and renewed, and lived her life happily and with focus. She felt satisfied and no longer suffered from the headaches that had become so common. When she had returned home, she had worked hard to change the diet of her entire family, improve the health of her husband and children, and teach friends and extended family how to find freedom through food. Alex had transformed into a health ambassador, so to speak.

Alex's before-and-after pictures received cheers and applause. She honestly did not look like the same person anymore. After answering a number of questions and offering some very practical recommendations to help children easily transition to a plant-based lifestyle, Alex concluded her speech and was met with a standing ovation.

I told the group I had faith that change was coming for each and every one of them. I hoped Alex's reveal had fostered the same belief in their hearts. I left the room to the sound of the immersionists talking about the talent show later that night and the preparations they needed to make for it.

DAY
FIVE

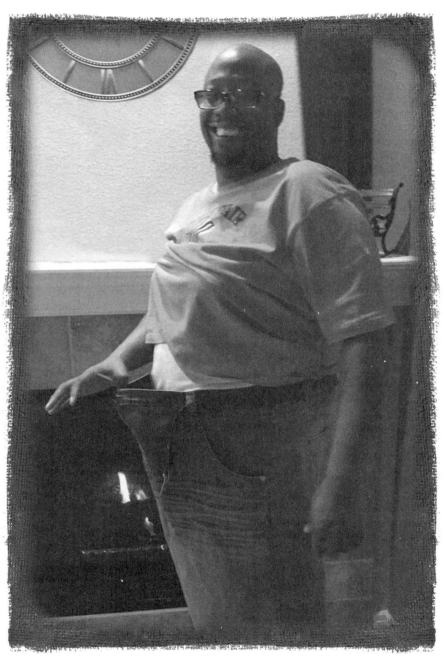

Milan finding a little extra room in his shorts after a few days of plant-based living.

*M*ilan's Story

I was awake by 5:15 AM on Day Five. I took a moment while still in bed to express my gratitude for all the wonderful things that had happened during the immersion week so far. I was looking forward to the day, and was particularly excited about the dinner cruise that evening. That's right. The immersionists would be cruising through the Gulf of Mexico while having dinner and watching the sun set.

Before I could enjoy the trip, however, I needed to get up and follow my plan for the morning. And my plan was simple. I wanted to walk on a treadmill for a full thirty minutes before the morning exercise class was scheduled to start. The night before, I had decided to set my alarm for 5:45 AM to ensure I would successfully meet my objective. By the time it went off, I had already taken my shower and gotten dressed. Michael had decided to sleep in, so I would be heading down to the gym alone. I switched off the alarm and walked out of my room, carrying my water bottle and exercise mat.

When I got to the gym, I quickly settled in on a treadmill. I told myself I was going to walk no less than thirty minutes, no matter what. Ever since the big volleyball game earlier in the week, I realized I could accomplish more than I'd thought I could. Before immersion, I would always look for any excuse to avoid exercising for more than a few minutes. The pain in my knees, my sore back, and the nerve damage in my thighs and feet all kept me from forging ahead in the past. I promised myself I wouldn't let any of those things slow me down anymore. I was determined to push through any discomfort.

At around 6:45 AM, I realized I had been walking on the treadmill for almost a full hour. I couldn't believe it. Sure, I was tired, hot, and sweaty, but I had kept moving. It suddenly occurred to me that maybe the only limitations I ever really had were self-imposed. I had once thought I couldn't give up coffee and still function, which turned out to be untrue. I had also told myself I couldn't exercise for any substantial length of time due to my physical limitations, but I had just done otherwise. I began to wonder what else I could do if only I put my mind to it.

At approximately ten minutes to 7 AM, I headed over to the morning yoga class being held on the beach. I arrived just before it started and saw my roommate Michael, who had saved me a great spot. He asked how my time in the gym had gone. I told him I had spent almost an hour on the treadmill and felt great. He smiled and said, "I wish I had gotten up and gone with you."

Michael and I parted ways after class and I went up to my room to shower and change before breakfast. One quick ten-minute shower later, I picked up the phone to call Iris and say good morning. I told her about my extended exercise time on the treadmill and the hour of yoga that followed. Iris remarked that something was definitely different about me. I expressed my newfound confidence in my abilities and explained how it gave me a sense of freedom I had not experienced in a very long time. After a few more minutes on the phone, we said our good-byes. It was almost 8:30 AM, so I went downstairs to have a good breakfast.

I entered the banquet hall and noticed there was no line for the buffet in sight. Apparently, my coming down to breakfast later than usual actually meant I could make my plate more quickly. I grabbed a bowl of homemade granola with almond milk, a couple of open-faced breakfast veggie pitas, an assortment of fresh fruit, and a green smoothie and made my way to my group's usual table. I sat down and someone mentioned that Michael had let it slip that I had been getting up early to get in some treadmill time before regularly scheduled exercise classes. Suddenly I was being asked if I was planning on doing the same thing again the next day. When I said yes, some members of the group asked if they could join me. I was surprised by their excitement to wake up earlier than necessary and get in some exercise before, well, exercising. I informed everyone that I didn't think there were enough treadmills to go around, but they didn't seem to care. They just wanted to give it a shot. "Meet me in the hotel gym at 5:45 AM tomorrow morning," I said.

After breakfast, Michael and I went to the ballroom to hear Dr. Stoll speak. His lecture dealt with the concept of dieting and the relationship between lifestyle and illness. He actually took us on an imaginary tour of the inside of the human body to give us a truly comprehensive understanding of lifestyle-related disease. Before immersion, had anyone told me I would be so utterly enthralled by a speech on the inner workings of the body, I would have laughed out loud. But all I wanted to do was listen and learn everything Dr. Stoll had to share. It helped that, besides being informative, Dr. Stoll also made his lectures fun.

During a quick ten-minute break from the lecture, many of us gathered on the patio. I had several people tell me they'd heard I was planning an exercise session before the actual morning exercise class the next day. I laughed and told them I was simply planning on using a treadmill. They asked if it would be okay if they joined me. Déjà vu! I smiled and said they were absolutely welcome to do so, but made it clear that this would not be a formal class or anything. No one seemed to care. The hotel gym truly wasn't that big, so now I was really worried there might not be enough room for everyone. I didn't have the heart to put out anyone's spark, though. *The more the merrier,* I thought.

I couldn't believe so many people were willing to give up sleep to join me in the hotel gym before we were all expected to attend regularly scheduled morning exercise classes. I realized something was definitely happening to all of us. We all seemed to be focused on taking back our lives in a way none of us had thought possible just a few short days before.

When the break ended everyone went back to their seats in the ballroom. Before Dr. Stoll continued, Tom took the stage and addressed the room. He informed us that we would need to meet in the hotel lobby at 4 PM sharp to board the buses that would take us to the dinner cruise. The whole room was buzzing at this announcement.

We couldn't wait. I even heard people discussing what they were going to wear. It was officially a big deal.

As Dr. Stoll spoke again, he explained how doctors receive only a few hours of instruction on the subject of nutrition while in medical school. I sat in my seat thinking how all my life I had assumed my doctor knew everything there was to know about health. It had not occurred to me that my personal physician might not have all the answers. I made a note in my immersion workbook that said, "My doctor is not all-knowing." This single bit of information was causing me to consider my healthcare in a whole new way.

After Dr. Stoll's lecture, everyone headed back out to the patio again for a little sunshine. While we stood there soaking it in, a few immersionists outside my regular group approached me and asked if our little gang was planning on meeting up on the patio after the cruise. "Yes," I said. They asked if they could join us. I found it strange that people were starting to look at me as the unofficial leader of this gathering. Since the talent show, however, people seemed to view me in a whole new light. I had gone from the funny fat guy to the man on a mission.

IT'S NOT UNUSUAL

Michael and I went to lunch right at 12:30 PM. It was no surprise that everyone in the banquet hall was talking about the upcoming cruise. We had all been wearing workout attire every day, so having to dress up a bit thrilled many of us. After having a quick bite to eat, Michael and I headed upstairs to our room. While Michael took a shower, I called home. Iris answered the phone and we chatted about the cruise. I told her I had brought a nice pair of slacks, dress shirt, and tie to wear. Before getting off the phone, I promised to take lots of pictures of the evening's festivities.

After about fifteen minutes, Michael emerged from the bathroom. I jokingly asked if he had saved me enough hot water for me to wet my entire body. After washing up, I grabbed my clothes to get dressed. Much to my surprise, my pants and shirt weren't really fitting right. Michael looked at me and said, "Milan, your outfit looks too big." I let him know that when I'd packed it five days ago, it fit just fine. He said, "Holy smokes! You look like you have lost some weight."

I stood there staring at myself in the full-length mirror. Michael was right. Both my pants and my shirt looked baggy. *There's no way I could have lost enough weight for this to happen in only five days,* I thought. Then another thought struck me. These were the only formal clothes I had brought; my other outfits were made up of T-shirts and either shorts or jogging pants. I quickly put on a pair of shorts and a T-shirt and headed down to the gift shop to see if I could find even slightly dressier attire.

Upon my arrival at immersion, I had a fifty-six-inch waist. I wore a "5XL" shirt—not the standard off-the-rack sizes you find in most stores. After a quick look around the gift shop, I managed to find a "3XL" shirt that actually looked like it might fit. I had gone down two shirt sizes in five days. On the other hand, I had no luck finding pants. I decided I would wear the casual beach shirt I had bought and a pair of pleated shorts that were now big on me. I would simply wear the shirt over the shorts and not tuck it in. So, instead of my original dressy shirt-and-tie look, I was now going for "cruisin' casual." As long as I kept my belt cinched tight, I knew my shorts would stay in place.

I went back to my room to change. Excited, I called Iris again to tell her what happened with my clothing situation. She asked me if I had weighed myself recently. I told her I hadn't since the day of my blood work. I assumed I hadn't noticed the weight loss because I had been wearing drawstring shorts everyday. Iris and I chatted for a few more minutes and then ended the conversation by saying we loved each other very much.

Michael and I went downstairs to catch a cooking demonstration before leaving for the cruise. The demonstration, once again led by chef Chad Sarno, focused on how to create great-tasting sauces, stews, and casseroles. Although the class was truly fascinating, I couldn't stop thinking about the fact that my clothes no longer fit me.

It felt impossible that I could have lost enough weight to warrant the purchase of new clothes, yet it was obvious that my old clothes were no longer the right size for me.

Once chef Sarno had wrapped up his demo, I approached the immersion staff physician, Dr. McGee, and asked if it was possible to lose a significant amount of weight in only five days, explaining what had happened in regard to my wardrobe. What she said left me speechless.

Evidently, when a person of my size changes his eating habits, as I had, it is not unusual to see double-digit weight loss in the first couple of weeks. Because I had cut dairy, salt, oil, and sugar from my diet, and had also added a steady dose of daily exercise to my routine, my body could release a significant amount of weight rather quickly. Dr. McGee said this effect would level off by week three or so. I was now curious about how much weight I had, in fact, lost, but it was time to head to the buses that would take us all to the dinner cruise.

THE CRUISE

When we arrived at the dock, everyone was so excited to see the yacht we would be boarding for the cruise. The vessel had two levels. The main level housed an indoor dining room and a great outdoor patio. The top level was completely open and had lots of seating. Although the weather had been a bit warm all week, on the night of the cruise Mother Nature had decided to give us a break.

The boat made its way out into the Gulf of Mexico and I could feel both the sun and the ocean breeze on my face. It was wonderful. I felt as though I was exactly where I was supposed to be. The only thing that could have made it even better would have been my family being there to share the moment with me. About an hour into the cruise, the staff began to serve dinner. The food spread was extraordinary. Everything had been beautifully prepared and laid out by the hotel chef and staff according to the instructions of the immersion team. There were lots of appetizers and several entrées from which to choose. There were also some very tasty-looking desserts.

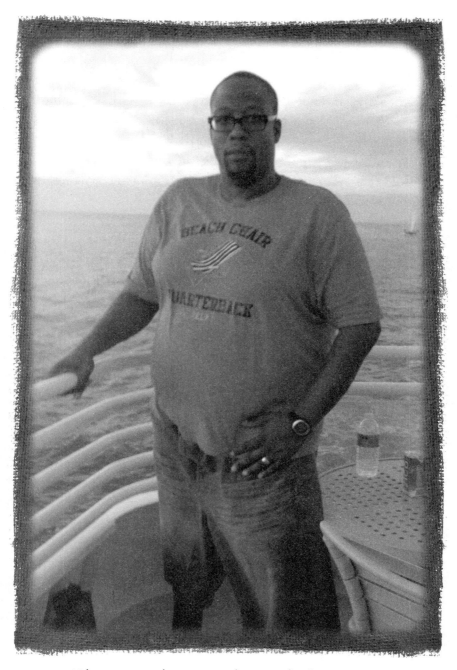

Milan enjoying the cruise and waiting for the sun to set.

I made myself a plate and then Michael and I settled in at one of the tables on the main deck, soon to be joined by our immersion family. As we sat and ate, we talked about how this entire experience had surprised us at every turn—from the quality of the food, to the fun of the talent show, and now to the amazing cruise. Dr. Stoll's Immersion was far exceeding all our expectations. While I sat there dining, I suddenly realized the people with whom I had been sharing this retreat were no longer just immersion friends, they were fast becoming real friends. I knew our common experience at immersion was creating a bond that would last.

After dinner, everyone moved up to the top deck to watch the sun set. While up there, we saw a large school of our buddies, the dolphins, following behind our boat in its wake. As the sun painted the cloudless blue sky, I thought about how far we had all come. I was actually beginning to feel a little sad that our journey was nearing its end. I knew we had only two days and one night left before we would all be heading back to our respective homes and families. Although I was excited to see Iris and Nigel again, I was still a little downhearted to recognize that in a few short days, my immersion experience in Naples, Florida, would be over.

The bus ride back to the hotel was full of laughter. Everyone seemed to be reaching their highest selves. When the buses pulled in front of the hotel, lots of people asked if there would be a patio party to cap off the night. What had started out as a few people hanging out on the oceanfront patio each night had unwittingly become a regular event. After the buses had emptied, there were more than thirty people mingling at our chosen spot. The laughter continued as we talked about everything we had been through over the last five days. We were having so much fun that we lost track of time. It was shortly after 1 AM when we finally called it a night.

Michael and I made it back to our room and quickly got ready for bed. I reminded him that there would likely be a bunch of people meeting us at the hotel gym at around 5:45 AM. After setting the alarm and scheduling a 5:15 AM wake up call, I quickly fell asleep.

$\mathcal{D}$r. Stoll's Story

The talent show the night before had us rolling in the aisles and wiping tears of joy from our eyes as some of the immersionists generously shared their amazing talents with the rest of the group. Milan had electrified the room with his poem "From a Keg to a Six-Pack," and I knew all in attendance had regarded his poem as prophetic. Seated at the back of the room, I had watched the show alongside my wife, and by its conclusion we had both received a boost of energy from the infectious spirit of the proceedings.

Drawing on the enthusiasm of the night before, I awoke on Day Five more excited than ever to speak to the group. I knew the day would be filled with important information that might require a degree of concentration to appreciate, so I was ecstatic that everyone seemed ready to receive it. I wanted to begin by tearing down an old mindset that frequently hindered successful change. I opened with a seemingly simple question.

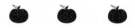

What does the word "diet" mean to you?

Think about that word for a moment and pay attention to all the ideas and emotions that come to mind. Just the mention of the word sends shivers up some people's spines. I want to help you redefine the word "diet" and remove your old mindset regarding the concept.

For you, perhaps the word "diet" conjures up thoughts of sacrifice, deprivation, cravings, and counting down the days until you can eat certain foods again. Maybe it causes you to recall dreaming about food, feeling frustrated and guilty, and consistently saying, "No pain, no gain." I would hope that such thoughts might make you realize how often a diet is a short-term plan with no long-term vision, that the real meaning of the word has been hijacked by a vast array of weight-loss programs, whose gimmicks have created a cloud of confusion that now looms over your food choices and body weight. With the existence of crazy diets like the "Cabbage soup diet," the "Grapefruit diet," and the "Morning banana diet," is there any wonder why so many are so confused?

The world has more diet books and dietary information at its disposal now than at any other time in history, and yet the global population is heavier than it has ever been, with epidemic levels of lifestyle-related diseases. It's enough to make one question if any diet ever really works at all.

MONEY FOR NOTHING AND YOUR POUNDS FOR FREE

A comprehensive Danish review of more than nine hundred studies on dieting from 1931–1999 evaluated the long-term success rate of dieting, which was determined to be a maintained weight loss of twenty to twenty-four pounds for at least five years.[1] It found that approximately 15 percent of dieters had kept the weight off by the five-year mark. Now consider this statistic: This year, a little over one hundred million Americans will go on a diet and contribute forty billion dollars to diet and diet-related industries. If the Danish review's analysis holds, then about ninety-one million people will spend their hard-earned money, as well as months of valuable energy and focus, on diets, but will not achieve long-term weight loss. Would you take on an extremely challenging project over the next two months if you knew it had such a slim chance of success? Most would not.

Why, then, do so many Americans take on new diets every year and hope for any better outcome? I have come to believe that the majority of people I work with are simply baffled by the tsunami of information that rushes toward them daily from websites, television, books, magazines, and neighborhood gossip. Most people find themselves making the same heartfelt wish every year—the wish that somehow this "shiny" new diet program will be the one that works for them. Instead, they should wish for clarity, which will lead to educated choices and permanent lifestyle change.

The origin of the word "diet" comes from the Greek term "diaita," which means "way of life." This is an inspiring definition, as it places food in its proper foundational position in life. Food then becomes an integral part of accomplishing your "why," your vision, and your passion. It rises above elementary ideas of convenience, taste, and pleasure to a new place of honor, respect, and planning. It encourages proactive decisions about what to eat.

Ultimately, your life should be energized by abundance and not constrained by scarcity. I have become convinced by the scientific literature and the changed lives of my patients that a plant-based diet of whole food is the key to eliminating the damaging ideas surrounding the word "diet" and replacing them with the notion of food as a way of life. Once you think of food in this way, I know you will find lasting freedom from lifestyle-related health conditions.

THE HEART OF THE MATTER

Have you ever wondered why so many people today develop heart disease, type 2 diabetes, or certain forms of cancer? The media often presents vague causal relationships to explain certain health conditions, such as the connection between cholesterol and heart disease, or how too much dietary sugar can lead to type 2 diabetes. But these generalized answers don't really help you understand the root cause of poor health, the contributing factors that allow the progression of a variety of diseases, or what you can do to prevent, suspend, or reverse some forms of illness. I would now like to discuss a few common degenerative diseases and investigate their root causes.

Heart disease is America's leading cause of death, affecting nearly one out of every two people during their lifetimes. Without a doubt, it will affect someone you know and love. Cardiologists and cardiothoracic surgeons, many of whom are my friends, work long days and nights to treat the physical consequences of this deadly disease, and in many cases they save lives. But wouldn't it be great if you and your loved ones never had to see a cardiologist to undergo a heart catheterization or coronary artery bypass surgery? Research tells us that it is possible to avoid such outcomes, and even in cases of severe disease, long and healthy lives may be achieved.

Earlier this week, I spoke about the progressive narrowing of coronary arteries, which supply oxygen-rich blood to the heart muscle. In short, over the course of a number of years, one unhealthy lifestyle choice after another can lead to plaque build-up inside your arteries. This accumulation of plaque, which is composed of various substances that include calcium, fat, cholesterol, cellular waste, and fibrin, understandably narrows arterial walls, cutting off optimal blood flow, just as mineral deposits in hard water can narrow the pipes in your house. The combination of plaque debris and poor blood flow often leads to the formation of a blood clot, which may then act like a plug in a narrowed coronary artery, cutting off its flow of blood to the heart completely. The heart muscle then becomes starved for oxygenated blood and sends emergency signals—crushing chest pain, sweating, shortness of breath, and possible pain in the left arm—at which point, medical care is necessary.

Treatment may include placement of a stent—a small mesh tube that opens up the blocked artery, allowing blood to flow. If there is blockage in multiple arteries, bypass surgery may be recommended. As its name suggests, this surgery bypasses diseased portions of arteries with veins taken from the inside of the leg, which are connected above and below the affected areas. Blood is then able to flow around these sections, saving the vulnerable heart muscle. Both treatments can save lives, but neither corrects the underlying root cause of heart disease, and research reveals that stents and surgical grafts can become blocked again after only six months.[2,3]

The good news is that there is a solution for heart disease, and as my good friend and world-class physician Dr. Caldwell Esselstyn likes to say, "If truth be known, coronary artery disease is a toothless paper tiger that need never ever exist, and if it does exist, it need never ever progress." Research shows us that the answer to heart disease is lifestyle. Remove stress, processed food, and animal products from your life and shift to a plant-based routine. To better understand this solution, we must take a look at the origins of lifestyle-related illness and the healing mechanisms inherent to a diet of nutritious whole food.

FANTASTIC VOYAGE

To get a clearer picture of the connection between lifestyle and illness, I would like you all to join me on a guided tour of the internal workings of the amazing human body. Our first stop is the front line of the battle for your health, where the fighting is fierce and the bullets are flying in all directions.

Maybe some of you have an idea about the part of the body to which I am referring, but you may be surprised. It's the brain. Your thoughts and beliefs about life and food happen here. It is where your choices concerning what to eat and what not to eat, how to interact with other people, how to organize your time and money, and how to deal with your emotions are made. It is the true front line of health and disease.

When you make a choice, it leads to visible external effects and less tangible internal effects. For example, if I choose to drink caffeine right before bed, I will toss and turn all night, feel tired in the morning, and have dark circles under my eyes all day. The internal effects of this choice will be less noticeable, though equally important. Not getting enough sleep will constrict blood vessels, increase inflammation, and produce a rapid heart rate.

Disease begins with decisions and emotions, which can deplete the resources and reserves of the body, affecting the immune system, hormonal system, and nervous system. In response to stress and ongoing demands made by the brain, the fight-or-flight system gets activated, the hormonal system increases production of the stress hormone cortisol, and the immune system goes into overdrive. These reactions create an environment in the body in which healing is impaired, genetic vulnerabilities are exposed, inflammation abounds, and illness begins to manifest.

Your choices may be influenced by your beliefs, relationships, history, emotions, or addictions. The decisions you make lead to actions in the physical realm. When your brain tells your arm and hand to pick up that box of cookies at the grocery store and eventually place those cookies in your mouth, it is giving that food access to your internal system and allowing the consequences of that choice.

From your hand to your mouth to your cells, the fantastic voyage of food is astoundingly complex, so in the interest of time, our little tour will stop at only the most important sites along the way. Now that we have looked at the brain, let's take a peek at the teeth and saliva in the mouth. Saliva contains enzymes, substances that accelerate chemical reactions. These enzymes begin the work of breaking down food while teeth grind through the indigestible cellulose walls of plants, exposing plant enzymes—such as the myrosinase in broccoli—to phytochemicals inside plant cells. This interaction activates the disease-fighting properties of phytochemicals. For example, phytochemicals in broccoli have been shown to fight cancer, reduce inflammation, and repair DNA.[4,5] Hopefully, this information will inspire you to chew your food a little longer in order to get those enzymes and phytochemicals working!

After chewing, it is a quick slide down the thin muscular tube known as the esophagus into the harsh environment of the stomach, where the real food demolition takes place. Powerful stomach acid breaks down food into smaller, more digestible packages. This strong acid is crucial for the activation of an enzyme called pepsin, which helps the body digest proteins. It is also required for the sterilization of the food and to assist in the absorption of minerals, including magnesium, calcium, and iron. Taking acid-blocking medication for acid reflux, however, can impair these vital processes.[6,7]

Our next stop is one of the most largely ignored sections of the body: the small intestine, which is actually one of the most active regions in the body. Once food leaves the stomach, it enters the small intestine, takes a sharp left turn past the gall bladder and liver on the right, and then loops around the pancreas, which we will revisit when we talk about diabetes. The combination of bile from the gall bladder and enzymes from the pancreas—a total of about eight cups every day—aids the transformation of food into even more absorbable elements.

The small intestine features finger-like projections known as intestinal villi protruding from its walls. These villi have cellular membrane protrusions known as microvilli, which form a structure that looks like a microscopic shag carpet and is called a brush border. This brush border is where absorption into the bloodstream takes place. Once the components of food enter the bloodstream, they first flow into the liver and are then exported to the heart through a vein, after which they are pumped to various regions of the body.

The tight connection between intestinal villi prevents absorption of any food particles that have not been reduced to the appropriate size and any substance that has been flagged by the immune system. Sometimes excessive protein in the diet, the use of pharmaceuticals, or substances such as gluten or dairy products can cause inflammation in this area of the gut, leading these tight spaces between villi to widen and become leaky. This resultant condition is known as leaky gut syndrome. Leaky gut syndrome allows larger food elements to access the bloodstream and trigger an immune response. This process has been recognized as a tipping point in autoimmune disease.[8]

Fortunately, leaky gut syndrome may be healed by removing irritating agents from the diet and boosting beneficial gut bacteria, as well as with the help of certain components of plant food, such as the flavanol quercetin, which may be found in onions, cilantro, and apples. The amino acid glutamine, which may be found in beans and greens such as cabbage and spinach, also assists in healing.

AN IMPORTANT LAYER

Before we move on from the small intestine, I want to briefly share with you a few facts regarding the journey these food particles take as they travel to cells throughout the body. All building blocks of food—whether that food is beans, carrots, peas, a candy bar, or a donut—exit the bloodstream and enter the organs of the body through a thin layer of cells within blood vessels. This layer is known as the endothelium. You have sixty thousand miles of blood vessels in your body. If you were to ball up this layer of endothelial cells, that ball would weigh the equivalent of your liver. If you were to spread this layer on the ground, it would cover the surface area of six tennis courts. The endothelial cells produce vital chemicals that protect and maintain proper function of blood vessels and surrounding tissue. Endothelial cell dysfunction has been associated with some of the most common illnesses, including heart disease, diabetes, cancer, asthma, Parkinson's disease, and autoimmune diseases such as lupus and multiple sclerosis.

One of the most important chemicals produced by endothelial cells is nitric oxide (NO). Nitric oxide resolves inflammation, prevents plaque build-up associated with hardening of the arteries, inhibits the formation of cancer cells, prevents blood clots, and causes relaxation of blood vessels, which reduces blood pressure. When endothelial cells become injured or dysfunctional, nitric oxide levels decrease. Low amounts of NO cause blood vessels to constrict, blood pressure to increase, blood platelets to become sticky and form blood clots, and, along with LDL cholesterol, plaque to form inside blood vessels. Moreover, the inflammation resulting from decreased NO levels may spread to other tissues, increasing the risk of cancer. Now that you understand how important endothelial cells are to your health, don't you want to know how to maintain a well-functioning endothelium and practically eliminate your risk of heart disease, the leading killer in America today?

Factors that harm endothelial cells will come as no real surprise: Consumption of saturated fats and trans fats, use of tobacco products, consumption of alcohol, consumption of too much sugar, elevated cholesterol levels, pesticides exposure, sedentary lifestyle, and stress.[9,10] In other words, our Western lifestyle and diet are detrimental to endothelial health, essentially injuring every system in our bodies. In fact, trans fats have been directly shown to increase risk of coronary heart disease, and the Institute of Medicine has declared that no amount of this substance may be considered safe.[11] Although many processed foods have been taking steps to remove trans fats from their ingredient lists, these fats occur naturally in animal fat, and so may be found in meat and dairy. A plant-based diet is the easiest and safest means of protection.

Endothelial cells produce abundant amounts of nitric oxide during exercise. Nitric oxide levels also increase after consumption of healthy fats, such as the omega-3 fatty acids found in walnuts. Moreover, the quality of nitric oxide is improved when exposed to phytochemicals, which only reinforces the benefits of eating more plants.[12,13] A diet of plant-based food optimizes endothelial cell function and has the potential to suspend or reverse disease.[14] In fact, Dr. Dean Ornish has documented heart disease reversal in his research. Using a plant-based diet, light exercise, and stress reduction, one of his studies showed a reversal of heart disease in 82 percent of participants.[15,16] When subjects were evaluated five years later, they displayed continued improvement and further regression of their heart conditions.[17]

Similarly, in a study of twenty-six individuals with advanced atherosclerosis, Dr. Esselstyn implemented a plant-based diet for the group and found that none of his subjects experienced any cardiac event over the next twelve years. After only five years, 70 percent of subjects showed regression of their atherosclerosis, and all participants had normal cholesterol levels.[18] Their narrowed arteries had opened up, cholesterol levels had plummeted, blood pressure had normalized, chest pain had resolved, and medications had been discontinued. These are powerful findings that offer great hope. Research strongly suggests that whole plant food optimizes function of the endothelium, reduces inflammation, halts further damage, and enhances the body's ability to heal and reverse lifestyle-related disease.

GOING WITH YOUR GUT

Now, if I may redirect your attention back to the larger gastrointestinal system, we can continue our tour of the human body. You may be shocked to find out that you have trillions of bacteria in your gastrointestinal tract, and you may be tempted to take something to kill that bacteria, as the mere suggestion of these little creatures probably makes you think of disease. While some of these microorganisms can be harmful, others are actually beneficial, even vital, to your well-being. A sufficient population of friendly bacteria—also known as probiotics—enhances the world of microorganisms known as the microbiome. Experts suggest that a healthy microbiome population is responsible for approximately 75 percent of the strength of the immune system.

Research has found that gut bacteria are involved in more processes than we ever imagined. They manufacture B vitamins and vitamin K, amino acids, and short-chain fatty acids, which help maintain blood sugar levels. They also aid in the breakdown of food, help produce the mood-related neurotransmitter serotonin, reduce inflammation, influence stress response, and even impact genetic expression. An adequate colony of beneficial gut bacteria might be one of the best defenses against disease.

So, where do all these important bacteria come from? The microbiome first springs to life at birth. During delivery, a baby acquires bacteria from its mother, in part through the vaginal birthing process. C-section babies lack this exposure, and thus may possess a very different bacterial population. Some research suggests these children may be more susceptible to conditions such as obesity, asthma, allergies, and autoimmune disease.[19]

Formula feeding and antibiotics may also harm a baby's new microbiome, putting it at risk for future illness. Nursing stimulates the release of bacteria from the mother's gut. These bacteria are infused into the milk and then transferred to the baby's developing microbiome.[20] Every time a baby nurses, bacteria from its mother colonize that baby's gut. Some sugars in mother's milk, once thought to be useless to newborns, have now been found to help feed the bacteria that form a healthy gut population in a growing infant.

Throughout life, the microbiome is influenced by a variety of factors, and the bacterial population is constantly changing based upon these outside influences. For instance, switching from a more plant-based diet to a high-fat, high-sugar diet can alter the type of bacteria in your gut, allowing a more sinister population to grow in just one day![21,22] Antibiotics, alcohol, stress, high protein intake, high sugar intake, and numerous medications are just a few of the things that can negatively affect the microbiome. But as you can see, most of these are part of the Western lifestyle, which has become known for its fast pace, high stress levels, and obsession with convenience and pleasure—the same lifestyle you will be leaving behind. Conversely, the resistant starches found in beans, lentils, and peas make excellent meals for good bacteria, while a type of fiber named inulin, which may be found in such foods as garlic, onions, and ripe bananas, may also be considered fine dining for microbes. Finally, fermented items like sauerkraut, kimchi, and pickles contain billions of live bacteria that may serve as new members of a healthy population.

Another perspective on bacteria may be seen in studies that have identified a link between high levels of dietary protein from animal sources and inflammation. Gut bacteria convert L-carnitine—an amino acid product found in very high amounts in red meat, but also in chicken, fish, and eggs—into trimethylamine *N*-oxide, or TMAO, a molecule that can cause inflammation. A growing number of studies have shown a strong association between meat consumption, higher levels of TMAO, and increased risk of heart disease and cancer.[23,24,25] People following a more plant-based diet have been found to have lower levels of TMAO, however, and a lower overall risk of heart disease.[26]

Let us now bring the tour to the last five feet of the gastrointestinal tract known as the large intestine, or colon, where water and vitamins are absorbed. The colon contains circular groups of muscles that move solid waste along through rhythmic contractions, squeezing it toward the exit at a rate of 1 centimeter every hour. This process is called peristalsis. If movement of waste is slowed or impaired, which can happen due to stress, inactivity, dehydration, side effects of medication, consumption of certain foods, or lack of fiber, stool begins to harden and accumulate, resulting in constipation.

The word constipation may bring back some traumatic memories of your grandma and grandpa talking about their bowel habits at the breakfast table, but constipation is important and has been associated with a number of significant diseases. The best defense is a good offense when it comes to constipation. Drink six to eight glasses of water a day, exercise and move more, eat fiber-rich plant food, stress less, avoid processed food and too many animal products, and work with your doctor to reduce your medications as you improve your health.

Sometimes the colon wall develops what appears to be a hole but is actually an outward pocket, or diverticulum. Diverticula were once thought to be created by increased pressure in the large intestine due to constipation caused by a low-fiber diet,[27] but now research is finding the problem to be more likely a result of degeneration of the nerves and muscle wall, as well as alterations in the microbiome.[28] The most effective prevention of diverticula is a healthy gastrointestinal system, which can be achieved by eating plant food, which is full of fiber and feeds good gut bacteria, as well as by specifically adding anti-inflammatory foods to your diet, such as greens, broccoli, or berries.

Irritable bowel disease has exploded on the scene globally as the Western diet continues to be exported to other countries.[29] While its direct cause is not entirely clear, it appears that genetic susceptibility may play a factor. This genetic vulnerability is exposed and negatively affected by dysfunctional gut bacteria, low-grade inflammation along the colon wall, dietary irritants and allergens, and altered motility.

The high-fat, high-sugar diet of our modern culture changes the microbiome, allowing overgrowth of sinister bacteria such as *Bacteroides* and a decrease in beneficial *Prevotella,* which is common to rural people and tribes.[30] These results create inflammation and irritation of the bowel wall. Other sources of potential irritation and inflammation to the bowel include various saturated fats, which are seen in high amounts in meat and dairy products, and omega-6 fatty acids, the main dietary source of which is most forms of vegetable oil. Sugar also increases risk of inflammatory bowel disease, while dairy and processed grain can irritate the bowel wall.[31] A large, colorful salad, on the other hand, is full of phytochemicals such as carotenoids, which can reduce systemic inflammation.[32] And as already mentioned, plant-based food contains fiber, which feeds the microbiome, while the cellulose of plant cell walls stimulate growth of colon wall cells, promoting healing.[33]

Before we finish our tour of the human body, I would like to point out that if we were to see a red growth extending into the colon like a big stalactite hanging from the ceiling of a cave, we would likely be looking at colon cancer. As this type of cancer grows and develops a blood supply, it can spread through local lymph nodes and blood vessels to other parts of the body in a process known as metastasis. Colorectal cancer is one of the most commonly diagnosed cancers of the digestive tract, but it could become a rare diagnosis with a change in lifestyle.

The Western diet has been linked to elevated levels of colorectal cancer. To shed light on this relationship, Harvard published the results of two large studies: The Nurses Health Study, which followed one hundred and twenty thousand nurses, and the Health Professionals Follow-Up Study, which followed fifty thousand men. The researchers discovered that consumption of processed and unprocessed red meat was associated with increased risk of dying of cancer or heart disease.[34] They also wrote in their conclusion, "Substitution of other healthy protein sources for red meat is associated with a lower mortality risk." These results were confirmed by a study of over half a million people aged fifty to seventy-one, which also showed an association between consumption of red meat and increased risk of dying of cancer or heart disease.[35]

You may be wondering what exactly is in red meat that increases cancer risk. Research suggests that as the human body absorbs too much "heme" iron, or iron from animal sources, both risk of cancer and risk of heart disease rise.[36,37,38] Research has also identified several other factors in animal products that increase cancer risk, including IGF-1 (insulin-like growth factor), Neu5Gc (N-glycolylneuraminic acid), omega-6 fatty acids, and endotoxins.[39,40,41]

Plant food, conversely, has several key components that have been shown to reduce colon cancer risk. In his study of the African populations, Dr. Denis Burkitt found that fiber reduces risk of colon cancer, a finding that was then strengthened by larger studies, including the largest European prospective investigation into cancer and nutrition.[42] But, as you now understand, it is not just one element that heals or harms; it is a combination effect that protects and renews us. Substances called phytates, which may be found in beans, nuts, seeds, and whole grains, have several powerful effects. They inhibit growth of cancer cells, cut off the blood supply to existing tumors, and cause cancer cells to return to their normal state.[43] The phytochemicals in foods such as whole grains, beets, broccoli, and the spice turmeric have anti-inflammatory effects, suppress cancer growth, starve cancer of nutrients and blood, and stimulate cancer cell death.[44,45,46]

Think of it this way: With each bite of a delectable plant-based breakfast, lunch, or dinner, you are protecting yourself against not only colon cancer but also the majority of lifestyle-related health conditions. Your daily diet is one of the most powerful, broad, and deep interventions to prevent illness available—and you don't need a doctor's prescription or even health insurance to start safeguarding your future today.

THE END OF THE TOUR

There is so much more to the story, but our tour must come to a close. It is probably for the best that we skipped the remainder of the journey through the colon. I am happy to have given you all a fun introduction into the formation and resolution of disease. Diet is one of the most crucial factors involved in the initiation and progression of disease, as well as in the prevention and reversal of disease. This is exciting news because it puts control back on your plate, so to speak. Instead of unknown causes, terrifying chemicals, or bad genetics looming over you and threatening illness, your daily diet, mindset, and lifestyle may play much bigger roles in the onset of common diseases. They can be powerful tools in the prevention or reversal of illness.

In the days to come, we will continue to look at the relationship between food and disease by highlighting other interesting areas of research. By the time you leave here, I know you will fight with every bite. Before I go, I would like to present you all with another affirmation.

Today I choose to respect and honor myself, my loved ones, and my future by choosing foods that heal my body, restore my health, and reverse disease.

That is all you need to take with you right now. I will see you all later on the cruise.

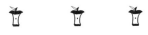

After an afternoon of understandable anticipation, our entire immersion family stood next to the three big yellow school buses that were waiting outside the hotel to take us to the *Naples Princess* sunset dinner cruise. In addition to offering a stunning view of the sunset over the Gulf of Mexico, the cruise promised an elegant evening celebration with a delicious multicourse meal, including my favorite three-bean chili and raw carrot cake. I told the immersionists we would not be discussing any internal organs on this particular tour. Instead, we would be treated to the sight of dolphins frolicking near the boat as we cruised through the canals and out into the Gulf.

DAY SIX

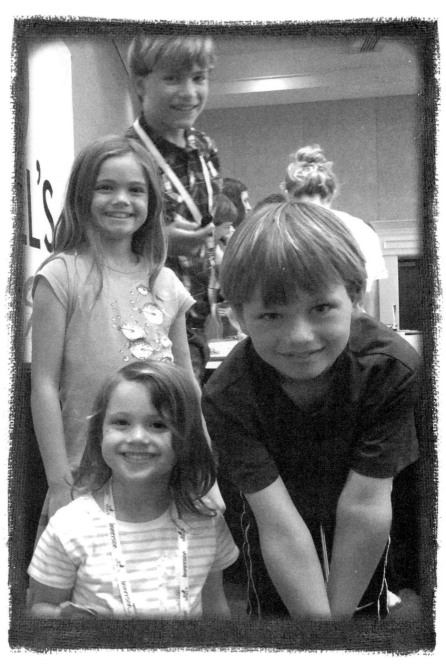

Dr. Stoll's children lending a helping hand at the family cooking demonstration.

$\mathcal{M}$ilan's Story

Day Six started off with a bang, literally. The vibration of my cell phone's alarm had caused the device to hop from the bedside table onto the floor. I had already woken up before the commotion, though, and had simply been lying quietly in bed, thinking about the fact that this day would be my last full day at the retreat. It was 5:15 AM. I quickly got out of bed and headed to the shower. Michael was still asleep. The night before, he had asked me to wake him when I was done with my morning routine.

When I emerged from the bathroom, I saw Michael had gotten up on his own steam and was grabbing his shower items to wash up. I told him I wanted to get over to the gym soon. What with all the talk of other attendees joining us for our morning workout, I felt the gym might get crowed early.

By 5:45 AM, Michael and I were heading toward the elevator. We both wondered if other immersionists would really show up at the gym, especially since we had all enjoyed a late night the day before. When the elevator doors opened, Michael and I saw over twenty people wearing their green immersion T-shirts and holding their water bottles. One of my fellow program participants looked at me and asked, "So, what's on the agenda this morning, Big Sexy?"

We were completely floored by the number of people who had shown up. After a quick head count, I realized there was no way all of us would fit in the hotel gym at the same time, considering there were already other hotel guests working out there. I turned to the group and asked, "Who's up for a morning walk?" Everyone agreed that a walk would be awesome, so we made our exit through the front door of the building and got to it.

That morning was much like most others in Florida, warm and humid. At least the sun had not yet come up and there was a bit of a breeze. I can only imagine what our group must have looked like to people driving down the street at the time. We had people of different races, cultures, and ages, and a great mix of both men and women. It was inspiring to me. The walk soon turned into a moving party. We talked and laughed amongst ourselves over the course of the entire trek. The combined energy of the group was palpable. Here it was, barely 6 AM and our caffeine-free walkers were fully awake, clear-headed, and keeping a pretty good pace, too. Everyone was motivated in a way none of us had been just six days earlier. We reached one of the nearby piers and stopped to take a few photographs, making our way back to the hotel soon after.

When we arrived back at the resort, everyone made plans to meet up on the patio after the big beach party scheduled for that night. That's right. Day Six would conclude with a beach party, complete with Tiki torches and a live band. This immersion was not only changing my life in ways I had never dreamed possible but also turning out to be a pretty amazing vacation. A quick check of my watch made me realize the walk had taken a little too long. We had already missed a significant portion of the morning exercise class. After chatting with the group for a few minutes, Michael told me he was going to head over to the class and take advantage of the remaining time. I decided to head up to my room and wash up before breakfast instead. In doing so, I could shower for longer than five minutes.

After a luxuriously long shower, I got dressed and then took a moment to call home. Iris picked up the phone and immediately said, "Good morning, sweetheart. I've missed you." I couldn't help but smile. I let her know I had been missing her as well. We talked about everything that had been going on with her. I then shared my morning walk experience with her. I was happy to have the time to talk to Iris for a long while. She said, "Milan, I am so very proud of you. I know that you are not the same person that left one week ago. I can hear the change in your voice when you speak. You have my full support." Although I was hundreds of miles away, I could feel her love. I told her I loved her, said good-bye, grabbed my immersion workbook, and went to breakfast.

I swiftly worked my way through the buffet line and then over to my favorite table. I sat down and looked around, noticing how transformed everyone seemed. We were no longer the disconnected ragtag bunch that had arrived just six days prior. Things were different and everyone knew it. We sat there and talked about our most treasured moments of the week, laughing and sharing in the same way a family does. Immersion had created a bond between us. We were having so much fun that we lost track of time (again) and almost made ourselves late for the first lecture of the day. One of our group pointed out that the speech was due to start in less than five minutes, at which point we all hastily gathered our belongings and headed to the ballroom.

GETTING MY FEET WET

In his lecture, Dr. Stoll provided a detailed analysis of type 2 diabetes, honing in on its causes, its complications, and the ways in which a plant-based diet may reverse insulin resistance and prevent this rampant condition in the first place. He also talked about the study of epigenetics, explaining the fact that outside forces could actually turn genes on or off. It was refreshing to hear that we are not simply victims of our genetics. Dr. Stoll led us all to rethink the idea of disease as a foregone conclusion of the cards we'd be dealt before birth. This revelation made me feel as though the power over my life had been shifted back into my own hands, or rather, that it had always been there.

When the lecture ended, we were given a ten-minute break, which many of us spent out on the patio, posing for pictures with new friends. It was obvious everyone was thinking about the next day, when we would all be leaving the retreat and reentering the real world. Each of us wanted to relish every last minute of this extraordinary experience.

After the break, we were treated to a cooking class hosted by Dr. Stoll and his wife, along with their older children. That's correct. Dr. Stoll and practically his entire family cooked onstage together. It was quite a cool sight to see. Witnessing this event helped me view meal preparation as something I could do with my own family. It suddenly occurred to me that if Iris and I were to include Nigel in the daily rituals of making breakfast, lunch, and dinner, he might just enjoy taking part. It would be nice to see him fully engaged in healthy habits that might follow him into adulthood.

The demonstration ended just before lunch. Everyone went to the banquet hall, where the atmosphere was starting to feel electric due to anticipation of the beach party scheduled for later that night. I thought it was utterly fitting that we would have a party. There was so much to celebrate. On a personal level, I was no longer addicted to caffeine and I had obviously lost some weight, but everyone in the banquet hall had something worthy of jubilant recognition.

After making my lunch plate, I met the rest of my immersion gang at our table. We spent the majority of our time laughing and talking rather than actually eating, it seemed. During all the shenanigans, someone mentioned the idea of taking a group photo during our final patio party later that night. Everyone agreed it had to happen.

I finished my lunch and decided to go for a barefoot walk on the beach by myself. With my sandals in hand, I started making my way down to the sand. I could smell the ocean saltwater in the air. The sand was hot, so I walked along the water's edge, ankle-deep in the ocean. With the sun on my face, I strolled leisurely, taking time to give thanks for the amazing opportunity to attend Dr. Stoll's Immersion program.

At 1:45 PM, I rejoined the immersionists in the ballroom, where a lecture by Dr. Michael Greger was starting. A world-renowned expert on clinical nutrition, *New York Times* best-selling author, and founding member of the American College of Lifestyle Medicine, Dr. Greger had a very entertaining way of delivering the facts. His speech dealt with the top fifteen causes of death in humans, which I thought would make for a humorless and dire lecture. I was wrong. The whole room laughed riotously as Dr. Greger made his way through the list, injecting a sense of lighthearted playfulness to the proceedings. As Dr. Stoll had also explained to us, Dr. Greger described how we might all save our lives by changing our lifestyles.

By the end of the lecture, it truly seemed as though living according to a healthy mindset could help anyone avoid most of the causes of death on the list.

After the speech, many of my fellow attendees met on the patio and discussed what the next steps on this journey might be. The real world felt as though it was inching closer and closer to us all. I listened as some people spoke of challenges they might face in getting their spouses or children to change their lifestyles as well. Others spoke about how excited they were to begin their new lives in earnest.

Late that afternoon, the entire retreat group met on the lawn for an official immersion group picture. Once the photo had been taken, all that was left on the schedule was dinner at 6:15 PM and the beach party at 7:45 PM. Having a little over an hour to kill before dinner, my patio family decided to meet at the hotel pool for a bit of fun in the sun and cooling off in the water. Michael and I returned to our room, put on our swimming trunks, and made our way poolside.

Our group played in the water like children. There were cannon-balls and back flips, games of chicken, and lots of splashing. I couldn't remember the last time I had been comfortable taking my shirt off to swim. Here I was, a forty-something man running around like a twenty-year-old kid.

As dinnertime crept ever closer, I decided to leave the pool gathering with enough time to head back to my room and shower before sitting down to enjoy my evening meal. I also took a few minutes to call Iris and Nigel and check in. Nigel answered the phone and asked, "Dad, are you skinny yet?" I laughed and replied, "I will find out tomorrow how much weight I have lost since arriving here, but yes, my son, I am definitely skinnier than I was when you last saw me." Nigel cheered in anticipation of seeing his "new" dad soon. I told him my transformation was just beginning. I still had a long way to go, but now I had a map to show me the way. Nigel promised to help me in any way he could. His sincerity almost brought tears to my eyes. I thanked my son.

Once Nigel had caught me up on all the latest regarding school and our family pets, I told him how much I loved him and asked to speak to his mom. Iris got on the line and proceeded to talk about her day. She told me that some of my coworkers had asked after me while she had been grocery shopping earlier. She also said she was ready to commit fully to the new lifestyle I would be bringing home with me. I couldn't thank her enough for being my rock. I let her know I was ready to come home. I had been missing her and Nigel dearly. After a brief but lovely conversation, I told Iris I adored her and would call her in the morning. Clean and revitalized from the shower, I put on a crisp pair of shorts and a fresh T-shirt and went down to meet Michael and the rest of the gang in the banquet hall.

CRAZY

As I stepped into the room, I immediately felt an enormous amount of energy radiating from my fellow immersionists. Everyone was ready to get his or her party on. This particular night's meal felt different from all the rest. It was as though I was meeting up with old friends for dinner and a great night on the town. Lots of people asked me whether there would be an unofficial after-party on the patio later. I quickly let them know there would be, and that all were welcome to come.

After eating another wonderful evening meal, Michael and I exited the hotel and stepped onto the beach to check out the set-up. As with everything else at the retreat, the beach party had been remark-ably arranged. There were tables with various types of fruit-infused water, chocolate-avocado pudding topped with strawberries, and other immersion-approved snacks. There were Tiki torches lining a huge area of the beach just twenty feet from the water's edge. At the far end of the festivities was a band, complete with stage lights and a sound system.

Michael and I surveyed the party grounds as the band began to play. It didn't take long before everyone was dancing and having a great time. Everyone seemed to be joining in, from Dr. Stoll and his entire family to the rest of the immersion staff and all the participants. I didn't see a single person standing on the sidelines. After a few songs, the band segued into "Electric Boogie," letting us all know it was time to do the "electric slide." We instinctively fell in line and began to dance in unison.

About an hour or so into the party, the band broke into Bob Marley's "Buffalo Soldier." Seeing the ball I was having and my obvious affection for the song, the singer invited me onstage to sing. I grabbed the microphone and let it rip. The entire crowd responded in applause. I hadn't felt so alive in a very long time. I was struck by the feeling that the crowd was clapping not only for me but also for themselves. We were all one. By the time we began forming a conga line, we had people who were not even associated with the program joining in.

While taking a water break, I was approached by a hotel guest who had not come to attend immersion. She asked if I knew where the bar was, looking to me as though she'd already had a few drinks inside the hotel. I explained to her that the party she was now at was actually an end-of-week bash for a wellness retreat, and that, as such, there was no alcohol available. She stared at me as though I had two heads and then asked, "If there's no alcohol, then why is everyone partying so hard?" I told her we were celebrating a new lease on life. She laughed and told me we were all crazy as she staggered off to find the oceanfront bar.

At around 8:45 PM, I was standing at one of the tables and talking to Michael and the gang when someone suggested we end the night by jumping into the ocean. Since we were standing only about twenty feet from the water and could hear the waves crashing onto the beach, we all smiled and contemplated the suggestion. After a few minutes of back-and-forth debate amongst the group, I looked at my new friends and said, "That's it! I am doing it!"

I started walking toward the ocean when all of a sudden the rest of the group ran up to me from behind. I stopped in my tracks as we all locked arms with one another and then ran toward the water. Before I knew it, we were in. Everyone cheered and laughed as the waves washed over us in the darkness of night. In a way, our collective leap into the ocean had been the final step of the immersion program. To all the other people at the beach party, we probably looked nuts, but to me and my extended patio family, that quick dip had meant a lot.

By the time we got out of the water, the beach party was coming to a close. The gang agreed to meet back on the patio in twenty minutes for our after-party. Michael and I headed up to our room to change. Fifteen minutes later we were sitting on the patio with what appeared to be more than half the immersion attendees. Apparently, word had gotten out about our tradition and no one wanted to miss out on the final informal get-together. During the after-party, the members of my core group got together and posed for a group photo. That picture hangs in my house to this day.

At approximately 1 AM, we all called it a night. Back in our room, Michael and I chatted for a few minutes about the night's events and all the amazing things we had experienced during our weeklong immersion program. We couldn't believe it was almost over. Michael mentioned how he felt as though he had known me his entire life. I told him I felt exactly the same way. We talked about our little immersion family and voiced our optimism about the future. We shot the breeze for a little while longer as we got ready for bed, and then we said our goodnights, set our wake-up call and alarms, shut off the lights, and went to sleep. Tomorrow we would be going home.

Dr. Stoll's Story

Before the first lecture of the day, I stopped by the kitchen to check in on the members of my family, who were preparing for the cooking demonstration we would be giving that afternoon. I opened the door to find my five-year-old son, Elijah, and my seven-year-old daughter, Joy, wearing prep gloves and rolling oat and raisin balls in their hands. They were also rotating their hips as though they were twirling hula hoops. I looked at my wife, who smiled at me in recognition of such a funny sight. She told me that the immersion chef had dropped by earlier and said that the best way to roll an oatmeal and raisin ball was all "in the hips." We laughed at how seriously our children were applying this advice.

I left my wife and children to their work and headed to the ballroom to give my lecture, which would continue the previous day's theme of lifestyle-related illness. I began by revisiting the subject of the digestive system, this time focusing on the pancreas.

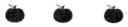

This morning I would like to return to our tour of the human body and take a closer look at the pancreas, so that we might address in greater detail the scourge known as type 2 diabetes. The pancreas is a yellow tongue-shaped organ that sits just behind the stomach. One of the most important duties of the pancreas is to control blood sugar levels. When you eat complex carbohydrates, which may be found in natural foods like grains, fruits, vegetables, and legumes, these nutrients are broken down into glucose—a simple form of sugar—which is then absorbed into the bloodstream. The pancreas responds to elevated blood glucose levels by secreting insulin, a hormone that acts as a key, opening the door to cells to allow glucose to enter. Once inside cells, glucose acts as biological fuel, providing cells with the energy they need to function.

Type 2 diabetes is a lifestyle-related disease that occurs when consistently elevated blood sugar levels and fat in muscle cells cause cells to become resistant to insulin. This resistance prevents the key from opening the door, forcing glucose to remain in the bloodstream. While type 2 diabetes is known as adult-onset diabetes due to the average age at which it appears, today this condition affects children as young as ten years old. In contrast, type 1 diabetes, or juvenile diabetes, occurs when the immune system mistakenly attacks and kills insulin-producing cells in the pancreas. As a result, type 1 diabetics require life-long insulin injections.

Elevated glucose levels can be determined in different ways. One common method is to measure fasting blood glucose, which refers to the amount of blood glucose after an eight-hour fast. Another method is to measure glycated hemoglobin, normally referred to as HbA1c, which indicates the average blood glucose level over a period of two to three months. Research has shown that risk of type 2 diabetes increases as these levels climb.[1] Additionally, in people with or without diabetes, risk of heart disease also increases along with rises in these measurements.[2] Needless to say, it is vitally important to identify the lifestyle-related causes of insulin resistance, as well as the steps we can take to reverse it.

Type 2 diabetes has been growing at near-epidemic rates across the globe. In the United States, the Centers for Disease Control and Prevention, or CDC, estimates that twenty-one million people live with a diagnosis of type 2 diabetes, while another eighty-six million are prediabetic, which means that their blood sugar levels are higher than normal, but not yet classifiable as diabetic. It is also thought that nine out of every ten prediabetics do not actually know they are at risk of full-blown diabetes.[3] If these trends continue, nearly one out of every three adults in the country will have type 2 diabetes by 2050. Globally, diabetes is projected to grow by 55 percent and affect 600 million people by 2035. Africa and the Middle East are forecasted to see increases in their diabetic populations of nearly 100 percent during that same time period.[4] Diabetes is costly both to people and nations, and if these numbers are correct, this disease will eventually touch nearly everyone in some way. I know there is a solution to this problem, however, and that these predictions do not have to come true.

Over time, elevated blood sugar levels can lead to nerve damage known as diabetic neuropathy, vision problems that include glaucoma and blindness, kidney failure, heart disease, and even cancer. The good news is that type 2 diabetes is largely preventable and reversible with a whole food, plant-based diet. But before we get ahead of ourselves, let's take a look at why cells become resistant to insulin. In so doing, we may better comprehend the reasons why a plant-based diet is recommended in connection with this problem.

NO JOKE

It may come as no surprise that eating refined sugar, processed food, and too many flour-based products is unhealthy, as doing so dumps excessive glucose into your system. But if insulin is available, why doesn't it unlock cells and escort glucose inside once type 2 diabetes has taken hold? The answer is actually pretty interesting. Research suggests that the fat inside skeletal muscle cells acts like tape placed over the "keyholes" of cells, preventing insulin from acting as a key to open their doors and allow glucose entry. Basically, glucose is left standing outside cellular doors.

While this information may be news to you, it is not a new finding. Research on this subject dating back to the 1920s found that insulin resistance rose sharply after a few days of a high-fat diet, exceeding any changes associated with a high-sugar, high-carbohydrate diet.[5] This finding has been confirmed by more recent studies, including imaging studies that traced fat into and out of muscles following dietary intakes of high-fat food.[6] In healthy subjects, a high-fat meal produced insulin resistance in just four hours.[7] Can you imagine how the body responds to the typical Western diet, which is comprised of more than 30 percent fat from meals such as a bacon and egg sandwich at breakfast, a ham and cheese sandwich with potato chips at lunch, and a cheese steak and fries at dinner?

It is not just dietary fat that contributes to fat-derived insulin resistance, though. Excess body fat pours free fatty acids back into the blood, escalating insulin resistance.[8] An overweight person can display insulin resistance that mimics that of a slimmer person who just ate a high-fat meal, even if that overweight individual just ate healthfully. This fact is even more troubling when you consider the typical Western diet, which spikes blood sugar and contains large amounts of saturated fat. This problematic combination can severely damage the delicate insulin-secreting cells in the pancreas, resulting in even higher insulin resistance and lower insulin availability.[9]

Excess body fat works against your health in so many ways. Although fat is often given cute names such as "spare tire," "love handles," or "beer belly," it is no joke. Over and over again, excess fat has been shown to increase disease risk. It is a factory that pumps out excess hormones and inflammatory molecules, activates pathways that lead to a pro-cancer environment, and causes excess wear on joints. Consider the fact that every ten pounds of excess body weight places thirty pounds of stress on the back and up to sixty pounds on the knees. Finally, the combination of excess weight and insulin resistance is not only the number one risk factor for diabetes but has also been linked to Alzheimer's disease.[10,11,12]

Fortunately, type 2 diabetes responds well to a plant-based diet. Studies that evaluated the prevalence of diabetes in different dietary groups, from omnivores to vegan, have found that vegans have a 78-percent lower overall risk of diabetes than omnivores.[13] A plant-based diet tends to produce bodies with less intramuscular fat compared to those of omnivores of similar weight. It also leads to improved insulin sensitivity.[14,15] In general, people who eat a plant-based diet for six months not only become healthier but also report higher levels of dietary satisfaction and control.[16]

Imagine for a moment the global media reaction to a pill that could reverse diabetes in the vast majority of people without any negative side effects. Such a treatment would dramatically change medicine, healthcare, business, and, most importantly, people and their families. Now understand that you don't need a prescription or medical appointment to get the same result. You can purchase your type 2 diabetes remedy in your grocery store today without significantly changing your monthly budget. This idea is not fiction; it is fact. Over three decades' worth of research prove it as such.

One study fed long-standing diabetics an all-you-can-eat diet of high-carbohydrate, high-fiber plant foods designed to keep body weight steady and eliminate weight loss as a factor in the outcome of the research. The study hoped to look at food choice alone as the primary intervention in type 2 diabetes. In just sixteen days, subjects experienced dramatic improvements and were able to reduce their insulin dosages significantly. Approximately 50 percent of participants were able to discontinue their insulin usage altogether.[17]

In a 1982 study, after twenty-six days of following the plant-based Pritikin diet and an exercise regimen, 87 percent of subjects were able to discontinue their oral medications and 77 percent discontinued insulin therapy.[18] Excluding exercise from the equation, a study funded by the National Institutes of Health pitted a vegan diet against the nationally recognized American Diabetic Association, or ADA, diet, which includes meat and dairy products. In every category measured, the vegan diet had better results: glycated hemoglobin readings were 70 percent lower, LDL cholesterol levels were 57 percent lower, subjects experienced 54 percent more weight loss, and 40 percent more medications were reduced or discontinued.[19]

Another study comparing a plant-based diet to the ADA diet went beyond looking merely at measurements of blood sugar, weight, and medication usage, and also analyzed changes in markers of inflammation and insulin resistance. The plant-based diet again led to greater improvements in blood sugar control, weight, medication usage, and insulin sensitivity. Perhaps the real hidden treasure of this research, however, was the fact that the plant-based diet reduced inflammation while the ADA diet had no effect.

This finding is significant when you consider the complications related to diabetes in which inflammation may play a key role, including heart disease, neuropathy, blindness, and cancer. Finally, the study's plant-based diet was associated with proper regulation of hormones such as leptin, which, as you know, stimulates hunger. This could be why reports filled out by both groups after the analysis suggested that the plant-based group has an easier time following its diet.

In terms of the possible consequences of type 2 diabetes, neuropathy, or nerve pain, and blindness can occur when damage to the small blood vessels reduces blood supply to fragile nerves in the legs, hands, or retina of the eye, resulting in local tissue harm and dysfunction. One study set out to determine if a vegan diet might provide any benefit beyond control of blood sugar for patients already suffering from neuropathy. Participants with painful neuropathy were placed on a plant-based diet and modest exercise regimen for twenty days. Remarkably, in four to sixteen days, 80 percent of subjects reported complete resolution of pain, improvement in numbness, reductions in insulin dosages, weight loss, and better cholesterol readings. Follow-up studies over the next four years revealed that 71 percent had remained on the diet and exercise regimen and reported continued relief from symptoms.[20]

In his profound research on diabetic retinopathy, Dr. Walter Kempner at Duke University placed diabetic patients with severe retinopathy on a plant-based diet of his creation, which included lots of rice and fruit. At the time of his study, no one had documented a reversal of retinopathy. Dr. Kempner used special photography to document any changes in his patients' eyes and then asked the head of the department of ophthalmology to review the photographs. After following the diet for approximately twenty-two months, thirteen out of the study's forty-four patients displayed improvements in both eyes, while seven subjects showed improvements in one eye —previously unheard of results in connection with diabetic retinopathy.[21] Exact reasons for these positive changes were not identified, but we can speculate from what we now know that endothelial cell function likely recovered, resulting in increased nitric oxide levels, better blood quality, healthier blood vessels, and reduced inflammatory molecules.

What I have presented today is only a brief summary of a few of the numerous studies that document the suspension or reversal of type 2 diabetes and its associated illnesses through adherence to a plant-based diet. Entire books have been written on the topic, but hopefully you can now see that the benefits of a plant-based diet go far beyond better blood sugar readings.

AN OUTDATED EXPRESSION

I would now like to share with you some emerging research that peers deeper into the body to present more thoroughly the profound impact of diet on genes and blood vessels, ultimately confirming the amazing health benefits of plant-based nutrition.

When babies are born, they represent pure potential. A newborn baby is an amazing combination of genes acquired from two individuals. Typically, when people hear the word "genes," they think of unalterable traits like hair color or eye color. This type of thinking has spilled over into ideas about common diseases such as heart disease, cancer, autoimmune disease, and type 2 diabetes. People often believe they are destined to get the same illnesses their parents had, but lifestyle diseases are not written in stone.

You are not cursed at the moment of your birth. These conditions are the result of external factors and everyday choices, which have the ability to turn genes on or off. The field of study that looks at the relationship between genes and the environment is called epigenetics, which means "above the genes." The science of epigenetics refers to changes in gene expression, which may be influenced by a number of factors, including lifestyle. In other words, choices you make in your daily life can affect whether or not certain genes become active or remain inactive. Research in this area suggests that your future health is tied directly to decisions you make today—what to eat, what to do, how to feel, and what to think. Power over your overall health has shifted from the health conditions you once thought simply to be the hand you were dealt at birth to the decisions you make each and every day.

The field of epigenetics was first discovered when researchers evaluated the birth weights of babies born during the Dutch famine of 1944, also known as the Dutch Hunger Winter. During the winter of 1944–1945, Nazi troops invaded Holland and cut off supply chains of fuel and food to four and a half million people in the Netherlands. Years later, researchers noticed a strange correlation while reviewing data of children born to mothers who had been pregnant during that time. Mothers who had been in their second or third trimesters over that winter had given birth to babies with overall lower birth weights and lower risks of disease later in life than those babies whose mothers had experienced the famine during their first trimesters only.[22] Depending on its duration, caloric restriction seemed to have resulted in long-lasting changes in offspring of this region at the time.

In relation to this research, a Swedish study discovered that the future health of children can be influenced by more than just their mothers. According to this study, boys who had experienced food shortages between the ages of nine and twelve were found to have grandchildren with increased life spans.[23] A striking conclusion from the literature on epigenetics is that a parent's life experiences and exposures are passed on to their children and grandchildren. Look at it as the power of choice multiplied. Your lifestyle will be an inheritance left to your lineage. This is truly an empowering thought for people starting families. You can help create healthy bodies for your children and grandchildren before they have even been conceived. This revelation will certainly create a more powerful "why" in the minds of many people.

Studies of twins have also documented the power of nutrition and lifestyle choices. Identical twins, who share the same DNA, can grow up to have different diseases and even height measurements. Differing environmental factors, including dietary habits, stress levels, and activity levels, turn areas of their genes on or off, either protecting against or encouraging illness. In regard to the majority of lifestyle-related diseases, the likelihood of both twins acquiring the same condition is less than 50 percent.

Further information in this area may be gleaned from research on Agouti mice. These genetically identical mice have a gene, the "agouti gene," which is turned on or off by diet and particular environmental exposure. One study showed that when agouti mice were fed a diet high in methyl groups, which are organic compounds that play a role in turning genes on or off, they acquired brown coats and lowered their overall risk of disease, while agouti mice that were fed a diet without methyl groups produced yellow coats, were obese, and had higher rates of diabetes and cancer. Thankfully, by simply changing the diets of pregnant agouti mice, coat color, weight, and disease rates of their offspring were altered.[24] When the fat, yellow mice were fed a diet high in methyl groups, they had small, brown, healthy babies that went on to live long lives.

Epigenetics is exciting because it means the diseases of today don't have to be the diseases of tomorrow. It would seem that the key ingredient to disease prevention and reversal is adding methyl groups to the epigenome through a process called methylation. This biochemical reaction occurs billions of times per second and plays an important role in DNA repair, sleep, mood, inflammation resolution, and the health of blood vessels. If the body does not contain sufficient methyl groups, these biochemical reactions falter and the person becomes susceptible to disease. So, what are the most abundant food sources of methyl groups? Investigators have found that leafy greens such as kale and bok choy, berries, broccoli, oranges, green tea leaves, sweet potatoes, apples, and soybeans are but a few of the plant foods that can protect your epigenome.[25] Simply put, a plant-based diet stabilizes and protects your genes.

Furthermore, epigenetic research recognizes that the most common diseases today—heart disease, type 2 diabetes, many cancers, osteoporosis, dementia, and lung disease—are related to lifestyle factors that subtract methyl groups from the body.[26] These factors include tobacco use, stress, and consumption of sugar, alcohol, caffeine, saturated fat, or salt. Fortunately, by eating plants, getting more rest, and exercising more often, you can add methyl groups to your body and protect yourself against these health conditions.

PUTTING THE PIECES TOGETHER

I would like to conclude this lecture by talking about the connection between lifestyle and cancer in particular. Cancer is a complex illness involving numerous contributing factors, both genetic and environmental, which initiate and fuel the abnormal growth of cells. Essentially, cancer occurs when certain cells lose the ability to undergo the normal process of cell death and instead continue to reproduce, forming tumors.

Time and time again, research has shown that the combination of a healthy lifestyle and plant-based diet may significantly reduce overall cancer risk.[27,28] The largest prospective study on cancer and nutrition tracked more than half a million people in ten different countries and found that four factors markedly reduced cancer risk: not smoking, maintaining a healthy body weight, exercising, and eating a predominantly plant-based diet.[29] It is important to recognize that prevention is the key to lowering cancer rates worldwide, and that diet and lifestyle lie at the core of prevention.

Although we do not yet understand all the ways in which food choices and lifestyle inhibit the growth of cancer, their effects on a natural process called angiogenesis may be involved. Angiogenesis refers to the formation of new blood vessels, which typically occurs when tissue is injured. The body responds to injury by growing new blood vessels to support healing. Once healing is complete, the body sends out chemicals known as angiogenesis inhibitors to stop further formation of blood vessels. In an unhealthy body, however, this process is disrupted, resulting in a dangerous overgrowth of blood vessels, which may be seen in connection with obesity, Alzheimer's disease, and cancerous tumors; or an inadequate growth of blood vessels, which has been linked to heart disease, macular degeneration, ulcers, and poor wound healing.[30]

Many studies suggest that factors such as inactivity, obesity, stress, tobacco use, overconsumption of sugar or saturated fat, and exposure to certain environmental toxins can alter angiogenesis, causing too much or too little blood vessel growth.[31,32,33,34] It would seem that if we were able to alter the angiogenesis process according to need, we might be able to stop a number of health conditions before they occur. For example, we might be able to prevent early tumors from quickly becoming life-threatening[35] by cutting off their blood supply with foods that suppress angiogenesis.

In regard to fighting disease through dietary choices, certain foods may inhibit the formation of blood vessels, potentially stemming the growth of cancer. They include leafy greens such as kale, chard, and dandelion greens, as well as broccoli, cauliflower, soybeans, berries, grapes, garlic, onions, turmeric, cinnamon, parsley, and mushrooms.[36,37,38] Sounds like a plant-based diet, doesn't it? In addition, stress reduction and increased exercise, which have been associated with lowering risk of heart disease and cancer, may also normalize angiogenesis.[39,40,41] While we still have much to learn about the link between diet, lifestyle, and illness, research on angiogenesis may simply provide one more piece of a very big puzzle.

By 2030, the developing world will account for approximately 70 percent of new cancer diagnoses.[42] We have exported the unhealthy Western lifestyle to people who don't have access to medical care. I must admit that this fact troubled me for months, and then I read a comment made by my friend and the founder of the Angiogenesis Foundation, Dr. William Li. He said, "For many people around the world, dietary cancer prevention may be the only practical solution, because not everyone can afford expensive end-stage cancer treatments, but everyone could benefit from a healthy diet based on local, sustainable, anti-angiogeneic crops."

Plant-based living can provide freedom from a number of health conditions to countless people around the world. As I look out upon the faces in this crowd, I know each of you will attain this freedom.

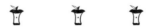

After my lecture, the hotel staff quickly transformed the stage into a kitchen for my family's cooking demonstration, which often ends up being one of the highlights of immersion for my family, as well as a favorite of many immersionists. I think it's important for people to see children involved in the process of preparing, serving, and enjoying healthy food.

My wife welcomed everyone to the temporary Stoll kitchen and shared her wish that this cooking demonstration would inspire people to see the kitchen as treasured space in which the family could grow and learn together. My older children assisted my wife in the preparation of healthy smoothies and then served them to the immersionists and my younger children. The revelation of the day, however, came when my wife made her sugar-free chocolate pudding. As the attendees tucked into their desserts, I heard someone in the crowd say, "If this is plant-based eating, then I can do this!"

DAY
SEVEN

Milan's Story

I woke up at 5 AM on the last day of immersion. I'd set my alarm to go off at 6:30 AM, but I was too excited to see Iris and Nigel later on, and too curious to find out how the readings from my second physical examination would compare with those of the first. The fact that my clothes were not fitting quite right anymore had me wondering exactly how much weight I had lost. The only events on the schedule were Dr. Stoll's parting lecture at 7 AM and the participants' physical reevaluations immediately following it. With no morning exercise class to attend, Michael had asked me to let him sleep in as late as possible.

I had promised myself I would get up every day and exercise, so today would be no exception. I grabbed my water bottle and headed down to the hotel gym, which was practically empty. I didn't see any of my fellow program attendees. I stepped onto a treadmill and allowed myself to get lost in thought as I walked.

I replayed the week over and over in my mind. So much had happened in such a short span of time. In seven days, Dr. Stoll's program had taught me a great deal, including the fact that I needed to let go of my guilt over what had occurred between my mother and me. It had also learned I was capable of doing a lot more than I thought I could do. Here I was, about to leave Florida, having achieved freedom from my food addictions. I could barely believe it. My daily rituals around caffeine consumption had been replaced by healthy habits. I hadn't eaten meat in a week and I really didn't miss it as much as I'd thought I might. Moreover, I had managed to exercise every day without fail during the retreat. I knew I had a lot more to be thankful for than just a paid week off from work. Despite my successes, however, I realized I still had a long way to go. My journey was not ending; it was beginning.

As I kept a decent pace on the treadmill, my mind began to focus on the steps I would soon be taking back into the real world. I felt slightly fearful of being challenged in ways I had not been during my week at the retreat. For the past seven days, all I had had to do was follow direction. The stresses of everyday life had been noticeably absent. I hadn't had to cook my own meals, clean up after myself, work at my job, or even make my bed. Everything had been taken care of for me. I knew my resolve would soon be tested once I returned home. Although I had not drunk a drop of coffee in days, I wondered how long my abstinence would last outside the hotel grounds, where there's a Starbucks on practically every corner.

Thankfully, I knew Iris would be there for me, supporting me as I continued on my journey. I couldn't wait to go home and share all the valuable information I had received at the lectures. I had made sure to take lots of detailed notes in my workbook, so that I would have the material at my fingertips when I needed a reminder. No matter what the scale might say today, I had experienced major personal growth thanks to the program, so I was ready to commit to it in real life.

At a little before 6:30 AM, I decided it was time to head back up to my room and take a shower before Dr. Stoll's last lecture. I also had to make sure Michael got out of bed in time for the scheduled speech. When I got there I was surprised to see that Michael had already gotten out of bed, washed up, and left. After showering, I called Iris and told her how excited I was to be coming home. She asked me if there was anything she could do to ease my transition. I asked her to purge our pantry and refrigerator of all the unhealthy things we had. Without hesitation, she said she would take care of it. With support like Iris, I knew I couldn't lose. I mentioned my upcoming final physical examination and promised to let her know how much weight I had lost as soon as I could.

THE MOMENT OF TRUTH

Heading downstairs for the final lecture, I was nervous at the thought of the physical examination I would receive afterward. I knew I had lost some weight and improved my blood pressure, but I was still worried about what the doctor might tell me. I had to remember that immersion was about more than reading test results. I had gained lifestyle skills and a new mindset, from which I would benefit for the rest of my life in countless ways.

I should have known that Dr. Stoll's farewell address would expertly touch upon many of the questions we all had now that we were leaving immersion. It was clear he was aware of the fear we were all feeling, and he took his time to provide sound advice on how to rejoin the world and maintain the change we had all experienced. He reminded us of the connection between lifestyle and illness, and how our reward centers work against us, encouraging food addictions that only a fresh outlook can beat. Hearing once again of the power of a plant-based diet really strengthened my resolve and made me feel confident in my ability to choose wisely going forward. I sensed I was truly letting go of my old mindset and permanently adopting one that would change my life for the better. Listening to Dr. Stoll speak, I knew I would be okay once I left the retreat. In fact, I couldn't wait to get home and start my new life.

As the lecture ended, I stood up and made my way to the testing area in the lobby. I checked in with the immersion staff and waited for my turn to be poked and prodded again. Before I knew it, I was heading behind a makeshift curtain to have my blood pressure taken by Dr. Stoll himself. It was 100 over 70, normal. I was thrilled to hear this reading had become typical for me. He then asked me to step onto the scale. I closed my eyes as I did so. The wait before hearing the number felt like forever. Dr. Stoll broke the tension by saying, "Wow." I opened my eyes and asked what he meant by that. He told me that, according to the measurements taken on Day Two, I had lost thirty-three pounds. He weighed me a second time, just to be sure. "Yes, you have lost thirty-three pounds," he said, recording the number in his log.

Without warning, tears of joy filled my eyes. I couldn't believe I had managed to lose thirty-three pounds. Dr. Stoll smiled and said, "Let's see how those lost pounds have affected your waistline." I stood there in disbelief as he began to measure my waist. "Wow again," he said as he checked my previous measurements. "Milan, you have reduced your waistline by six inches." I broke down completely and cried. I hugged him and let him know how thankful I was to him and his whole family.

When I emerged from the curtain, I saw lots of immersion participants in the testing area. A few of them asked me, "What were your numbers?" I revealed my results and was immediately brought into a congratulatory group hug. It was an extremely moving moment, but all I could think about was calling Iris and sharing the news with her. I decided to pop back up to my room and call her before going to breakfast.

She answered the phone and I was so anxious I could barely get the words out of my mouth properly. "Baby, you are never going to believe what I just found out. I lost thirty-three pounds and six inches." Iris asked me to repeat what I had just said, which I was happy to do. "Wow," she said. I was getting used to hearing that word. "I am so proud of you. I knew this week was going to be special for you." Iris and I talked about the future, our family, and how we would embrace this new lifestyle together. Hearing her voice made me anticipate seeing her beautiful face again even more. I was ready to go home. First, however, I had to go to breakfast.

I entered the banquet hall and was soon greeted by Michael's wonderful grin and the other smiling faces of my extended immersion family at its normal table. I sat down and shared my test results with everyone. Michael said he knew my numbers were going to be big. I asked if anyone else would be willing to reveal his or her results and was happy to see a bunch of hands go up. We'd obviously grown close enough that no one felt bashful to be honest. We went around the table and heard each person's story. By the end of it all, I was close to tears again. Everyone had changed for the better, whether that change was reflected in pounds lost, renewed emotional well-being, or a transformed mindset. I knew I would think of these people whenever I needed to regain clarity of purpose in my life from now on.

We all exchanged phone numbers, took some group photos, and basically took our time. There was nothing left for us to do but enjoy each other's company. At around 9:30 AM, a few members of our troop started to discuss going swimming one last time before we all left. The rest of us immediately chimed in and said it was a great idea. After changing into our bathing suits, we spent the remainder of the morning at the pool, laughing, chatting, and relaxing together. It felt as though we were simply on vacation.

Our pool party came to an end at around noon, as we all returned to our rooms to change for lunch. I took a fast shower, and then Michael and I chatted as we packed our suitcases. We made plans to see each other again soon, but admitted how excited we were to see each other off on our respective journeys. I knew Michael and I would remain friends long after immersion.

We walked into the banquet hall and couldn't help but feel a tremendously strong bond between the people in the room. There were lots of hugs and good-byes, and, of course, great food. Before I knew it, lunch was over. Michael and I went back upstairs one last time, grabbed our suitcases, and headed down to the lobby, which was full of immersion staff and participants waiting for the shuttles that would take us to the airport.

I couldn't help but think of my first day at the hotel. I could never have predicted the amount of weight I would end up losing. Even during the week, the only real evidence of weight loss had been the fact that my clothing had begun to fit me a little loosely. I hadn't really seen a big difference in my body size just yet. What I had seen, however, was someone who had started to believe he was in control of his life. Over the years, I had abandoned the idea of taking care of myself, leaving that responsibility in the hands of my doctors. Obviously, that approach had not been working.

I now had the answers I required and knew it was time to be the person I'd been hoping to be for so long—the person I needed to be for my wife, my child, and myself. As these thoughts played in my mind, I heard one of the immersion staff members announce that we would be boarding the shuttles in a few minutes.

THE REAL WORLD

We arrived at the airport and the real world dawned on us. We were soon inundated with a plethora of bad food and drink choices. The sights and smells we had left behind were now front and center. After getting settled in at my flight gate, I called Iris to check in. Iris confirmed my pick-up time and we talked about all the junk food I now had to confront. I told her that, even though it all smelled good, I had no desire to eat any of it. I didn't even want to get a cup of coffee. I explained that I wanted to continue my journey by getting up every morning and working out before breakfast, and she agreed to join me. I couldn't wait to see her and Nigel.

As I sat there waiting to board the plane, I began to notice all the crazy food products people were eating. It seemed as though I was being tested right out of the gate. Now that I was living a healthy lifestyle, I couldn't help but see everyone around me doing the exact opposite. People were eating candy bars and chips, drinking sodas and large cups of coffee, and buying lots and lots of fast food. I placed my earbuds in my ears and tried to relax with a bit of music. The real world was not going to coddle me.

When my plane arrived in Denver, I disembarked the aircraft as fast as I could and got my suitcase from baggage claim. When I saw Iris and Nigel pull up in the car outside arrivals, I almost jumped with excitement. Iris stepped out of the vehicle and proceeded to plant a big kiss on me. Then I opened the back door of the car and kissed and hugged Nigel. He immediately asked me how much weight I had lost. I told him I'd lost a little over half of what he weighed. I put my suitcase in the trunk, hopped into the driver seat, and started the journey home. Out of the corner of my eye, I could see Iris staring at me. I glanced at her and smiled. She said, "Wow, Milan. You can really tell you've lost some weight, especially in your face." Nigel then said jokingly, "Dad, you don't have a fat head anymore." We all laughed aloud.

After arriving at the house and setting my bag down, I asked Nigel and Iris to join me on the couch. We sat closely as I shared the details of my immersion experience. Iris mentioned the fact that she had already picked up the ingredients for a healthy dinner recipe she'd found, so the three of us spent the rest of the evening preparing a nice meal together. The next day we would go grocery shopping and restock the house with real food.

*D*r. Stoll's Story

The palm tree-lined Gulf Shore Boulevard was deserted except for the occasional passing golf cart. It was still early in the morning—the last one of immersion—and I was taking a sidewalk stroll to clear my head. As I turned and headed back to the hotel, my steps kept pace with the steel drum music still resonating in my mind from the beach party the night before. What a beautiful celebration of life it had been. Many attendees had worn their green "I survived Dr. Stoll's Immersion" T-shirts for the occasion. Having taken place just steps from the ocean, the shindig had even inspired part of the group, including Milan, to take a nighttime dip in the warm Gulf waters. The happy, rhythmic island music had brought everyone to their feet, dancing and doing the limbo, for which my youngest son, Elijah, had displayed remarkable skill, delighting the immersionists.

During the festivities, a participant named Ted had approached me and said, "Doctor Stoll, before I came to immersion, I felt I was done physically, mentally, emotionally, and spiritually, and I didn't know how I was going to get out of bed every day and support my family. Now I feel alive, more alive than I've felt in decades. My pain is gone. I am full of hope for my life and energy to take care of my family. This experience has been life-altering. Thank you, and please thank your entire staff for me." I don't think I could have asked for a better finale to my seventh immersion.

I entered the hotel ballroom to find the previous night's party hadn't really stopped. The immersionists were laughing, engrossed in spirited conversation, and seemingly enjoying just being in the moment. The contrast between the first day of the retreat and the last day was all the evidence anyone might need to support the adoption of a lifestyle based on eating a whole food, plant-based diet and getting regular exercise. It clearly changed lives in one week. I stepped onstage to address the group as a whole for the last time before they would all return to their homes and regular lives. Mindful of the attendees' upcoming transition, I always use my final speech to answer the questions that most commonly remain at the end of every immersion.

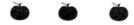

Good morning, everyone. Seeing you all this morning with bright eyes and warm smiles reinforces the amazing potential of just one week of plant-based meals and regular exercise. Isn't it incredible to know that it is possible to change the course of your life in only seven days? Congratulations on overcoming the challenges of food withdrawal, sore muscles, new tastes and foods, unfamiliar faces, new information, and caffeine-free mornings. Of course, let's not forget your new and improved bowel habits; I'm sure your roommates haven't!

I would like to take some time to talk about the fact that you will be stepping back into the real world very soon. You have all learned and experienced so much this week that none of you will be returning to everyday life as the same person you once were. You now understand the power of plant-based food to prevent, suspend, or reverse some of the most common diseases today, including heart disease and type 2 diabetes. You know the ways in which sugar, fat, and salt stimulate reward centers in the brain and motivate you to eat more and more unhealthy food over time. You have learned that a plant-based diet can stabilize hunger signals and leave you feeling full and satisfied at the end of every meal. You are aware of the significant influence the microbiome has on your immune system, and that a plant-based lifestyle is the best method of maintaining healthy gut bacteria. Finally, you recognize that emotions such as stress are tied to food choices and impact your overall health, and that through forgiveness, gratitude, and love, you can break free from their hold on you.

You have let go of old mindsets and established new, empowering beliefs about yourself and the world around you. You know your "why," you have learned to speak words of positivity to yourself and others, and you now see the wonderful gift of choice each new day presents. What a week.

Despite all this new information now at your disposal, I have no doubt many of you have questions you'd like answered before you get on those return flights home. I must admit, I hear the same concerns at the end of every retreat, and they are all very valid and worth discussing.

Before we get to these questions, though, I'd like to address a particular inquiry each of you will no doubt receive at some point in the real world, which is, "If you don't eat meat or dairy, how do you get the calcium, protein, and vitamin B_{12} your body needs to function properly?" When you hear this question—and you will hear it, I assure you—remember that a well-balanced plant-based diet provides the body with more than enough protein. If you consume a sufficient amount of calories from protein-rich plant sources such as beans and lentils, then you will meet your daily protein requirements easily. Similarly, a plant-based diet that includes soy beans, tofu, and leafy greens such as kale, bok choy, Chinese cabbage, broccoli, collard greens, okra, and mustard greens yields enough calcium for the body to maintain adequate bone density.[1,2] In fact, one cup of collard greens provides the same amount of calcium as one cup of milk, and a well-balanced vegan diet commonly contains 1,000 mg to 1,500 mg of calcium every day. Moreover, numerous types of nondairy milk are fortified with calcium and widely available.

As for vitamin B_{12}, yes, it is necessary to supplement your diet with this nutrient if you are following a plant-based lifestyle, although I would recommend doing so for anyone, as some research suggests that meat-eaters are actually more likely to be deficient in vitamin B_{12}. Vitamin B_{12} comes from bacteria, and our ancestors, as well as their livestock, got enough of this vitamin simply by eating food from the ground that was still dirty. These days, the food supply has essentially been sterilized, making supplementation with vitamin B$_{12}$ a good idea. I recommend taking 2,500 mcg of cyanocobalamin, a form of vitamin B$_{12}$, once a week. For people over the age of sixty-five, it may be necessary to take 1,000 mcg every day, due to an age-dependent reduction in absorption.

Now that we've answered the questions you are likely to hear, let me discuss the questions each of you are asking yourself at this point. I am willing to bet that you are wondering how you are ever going to maintain this new lifestyle in a world that doesn't provide much support for it. I believe it is important to remember your "why," and the way in which your health is connected to it. Doing so will help you maintain clarity of vision in regard to your health. As much as possible, surround yourself with supportive, encouraging friends that believe in you and your vision. When you get home, I would encourage you to call or text your friends and ask them to help you in your change. You will soon find out who your supportive friends are. Every once in a while, send a picture of one of your healthy meals to your supportive friends via text or email. Chances are you will receive positive words in response, which will boost your sense of commitment. Try to celebrate your successes with others as much as you can. A good social network is crucial to your new mindset.

Stay in touch with your emotional self. Don't allow food to be a temporary pacifier. Seek out meaningful and sustainable solutions instead. Finally, remember to be your own cheerleader. Identify and remove all negative thoughts from your mind as best you can, and put an end to all hurtful internal monologues as soon as you recognize them as such.

Knowing the power of a plant-based lifestyle, you might be excited to help close family members adopt this new mindset along with you, but unsure how to go about doing so. It is important to remember that you have had an entire week of immersion, but your family has not. Be patient with them, make slow changes, and educate them in small doses. Mostly, lead by example. Live a healthy life and others will notice and want to join you without having to be prodded. Don't let food become divisive. Healthy food should draw us together and ultimately heal relationships, not hurt them.

If you are working with your children, one of the best suggestions I can give you is to remove unhealthy foods from your home, that way you will avoid arguments over how much and how often these foods may be consumed. If it is not in the house, it won't be an issue. When poor food choices are unavailable, you can give your children the freedom to access the refrigerator and pantry without any restrictions. In turn, they will learn how to make healthy food choices on their own and achieve well-being independently. Do not be the food police. Your goal should be to raise wise, self-governing children who have the information to reach the best decisions possible.

Make your children a meaningful part of meal planning and take this time to teach them what you have learned. Take them grocery shopping and look though cookbooks with them. Get them involved, even in clean-up. Lead your children into health through love and passion, and avoid using fear, food rewards, or guilt as motivators. Find things in their lives that most affect them—for instance, a teenager may want to get rid of acne—and teach them how food can improve those aspects of their lives. Moreover, have fun and make this area of life an exciting adventure by trying interesting meals and healthy desserts, and using your kitchen to promote happy lives.

Speaking of family, most immersionists worry about how they might end up eating over the holidays or at get-togethers. During these types of celebrations, you can offer to bring food to contribute to the meal. Most hosts would be grateful for your generosity, and you will also be creating an opportunity for others to experience delicious plant-based dishes. You may find that people have questions about your diet. When you explain it, give only a bit of intriguing information at one time and let them consider it as they see fit. Don't overwhelm them. If they are still curious, they will follow up. In this way, you set up a positive conversation. If you are not able to provide your own food, keep in mind that these occasions are temporary, so just do your best to lead with love and grace, and remember to reset yourself with a good green smoothie in the morning.

Of course, many of these questions are actually just variations on the real question: How do I not fall off the wagon? First, please do not go about your life in constant fear of failure. Instead, speak words of success to yourself each morning. This is a process of improving your diet and health, not a success or failure proposition. Remember, it is all about making the best next choice. Achieve a healthy lifestyle one step or meal at a time. If you can, find someone who is familiar with your situation, someone who has been there, perhaps someone from immersion, who can help you stay on track and regularly encourage your new mindset. This type of support will be incredibly powerful in the coming months. Review your notes, read a book on the topic of plant-based eating, purchase documentaries on healthy living and watch them when you need to be inspired, or cut out pictures of your dreams and goals and place them where they will be seen during your daily activities.

When you get home, develop a menu for the week and then go shopping for the ingredients, making certain to fill up your refrigerator with wholesome plant-based food. As I mentioned earlier, remove all tempting junk food from your home. Doing so will not only ensure your family gets healthy meals consistently but should also keep you from reverting back to old habits. You might also learn to prepare a few delicious snacks, like kale chips or hummus and vegetables, and make them available when you're feeling vulnerable. If you are going to have a sweet dessert, have it at a restaurant or café, but don't purchase it to bring home.

Finally, buy a few cookbooks that contain delicious-sounding plant-based dishes. Commit to trying these new recipes, and allow for the fact that new meals don't always turn out well or taste as good as you'd thought they would. That's just the price of discovering new enjoyable recipes and building your own healthy repertoire of dishes.

Now, as much as I'm sure we'd all love to stay at this lovely hotel indefinitely, the reality is that we will all be returning to our busy daily grinds later this afternoon. So, how can you make this new mindset mesh with a busy schedule? The answer is planning. I have found that with a little preparation, a plant-based lifestyle can fit into even the busiest schedule. Generally, I recommend getting your breakfast as close to made as you can before you go to bed. Put kale, frozen berries, water, and a banana or frozen mango in a container in the fridge at night and then throw these items into a blender in the morning to make a smoothie in thirty seconds. Place a pan on the stove and have a portion of steel-cut oats on the counter nearby, ready to be covered in water and heated up in the pan as soon as you wake up. And don't forget your crock-pot, if you have one. In your crock-pot you can slowly cook cinnamon, apples, and steel-cut oats covered in water overnight and awaken to a beautiful bowl of healthy goodness. Of course, crock-pots are great for making dinner as well, and there is no shortage of plant-based recipes available for your slow cooker.

Cooking in batches on the weekend is an efficient method of preparing numerous servings of whole food, plant-based soups, stews, or casseroles and freezing them to be quickly defrosted and ready to eat at almost any time throughout the week. You may also want to chop up a variety of vegetables and keep them individually in covered containers. These veggies can be thrown on top of chopped lettuce for a nice salad in no time. I would also encourage you to make your lunch while you are cleaning up dinner. Put some leftovers in a Tupperware for your next afternoon meal and you're done, or prepare a veggie wrap with hummus and stick it in the refrigerator.

Remember that you are investing in your present and your future with food you choose today, as it affects how you feel today and will significantly impact your health in the years to come.

Although you are returning to a world that does not yet embrace the importance of following a whole food, plant-based lifestyle, you are also returning a different person than you were before this retreat. You have seen and experienced the transformational power of the right mindset. That which you have learned you cannot unlearn. It will be with you always.

Thank you all for an incredible week. It has been my honor to spend immersion with each of you, and I cannot wait to hear your personal stories of change in the near future.

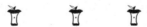

The group exited the ballroom and headed toward a cordoned-off area of the lobby, where each immersionist would have his or her blood taken and undergo a brief physical examination, the results of which would be compared with readings from earlier in the week. I was happy to see the first person to sit at my table was Milan. With his "Big Sexy" nametag dangling over his green "I survived Dr. Stoll's Immersion" T-shirt, Milan smiled at me and said, "Doctor Stoll, I can't believe it. I feel like a different person. This immersion was the answer I'd been praying for, Doc. I can't thank you enough."

I reached for my stethoscope and blood pressure cuff, anticipating the sharp pain in my elbow I'd felt while performing these examinations the first time. Thankfully, I discovered my elbow no longer hurt, and I was able to pump up the cuff without experiencing any pain. *Yet another benefit of a plant-based diet,* I thought: *a speedy recovery from injury.*

"Your blood pressure is normal," I told Milan. I could see he was relieved to hear it. When I told him his weight and waistline, he was overwhelmed. He had lost thirty-three pounds in one week. In doing so, he had also shed six inches from his waistline. Even I was impressed, and I'd thought I'd seen it all. Milan gave me a big hug. With his arm around my shoulder, he said, "I am going to keep in touch with you between now and the next immersion, because you know I'll be back as a reveal." I laughed and told him I looked forward to it. Although Milan had certainly changed, he was still Milan.

One by one, immersionists left the examination area in tears of joy and gratitude. When it was all over, I sat there for a few moments and took a few deep breaths. I couldn't help but smile. I carefully packed my stethoscope and blood pressure cuff and made my way to the banquet hall for the final breakfast buffet—one more big bowl of my favorite blackberries. My family awaited me at one of the tables, and as I entered the room my youngest daughter, Faith, ran to me and leapt into my arms, pointing the way to my seat. After breakfast, my family and I walked around the room and said our good-byes to each attendee.

Before long, I realized we had just a couple of hours to pack up and drive to the airport. Beyond the perfect weather we'd enjoyed over the last seven days or the breathtaking location at which we'd spent the entire week, in my heart I had a feeling this immersion had been a very special one—one that would continue to act as a source of inspiration to all those who had experienced it.

THE
CHANGE

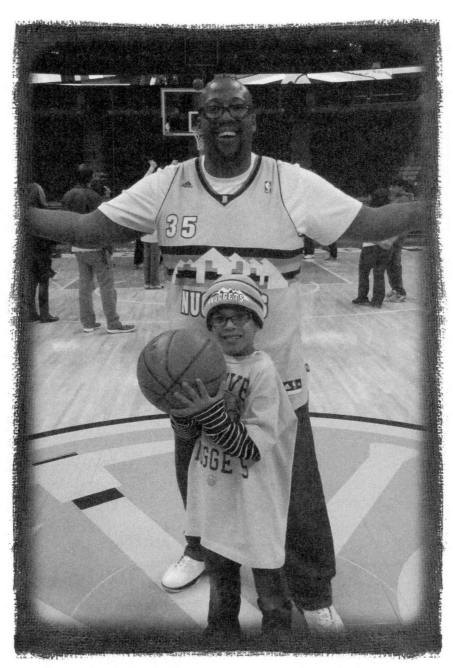

Milan back in Colorado, continuing his change.

*M*ilan's Story

When I originally made the decision to attend Dr. Stoll's Immersion program, I did so out of desperation. I felt as though I had already tried everything else, and none of it had worked. Before attending the retreat, I had lost weight a number of times, but had also gained it back each time. I must have tried every new piece of exercise equipment available, believing slogans like, "Radically change your body in just five minutes a day!" I had also bought every miracle diet pill advertised on late-night TV. And don't even get me started on all the fad diets I had tried. Looking back, I realize all the gadgets, pills, and diets over the years were simply the means for me to feel, even if for the briefest of moments, hope—hope that one day my life and health would improve. Back then, I would have done anything not to feel so hopeless. I would wake up each day to the thought that my body was more than likely going to be my tomb. I felt trapped in the form I had created and saw no escape.

I believed I had done so much harm to my body that it could not possibly recover from the damage. At best, I thought it would take two lifetimes to see any positive results from a change in lifestyle. I wished I could take my son to the park and play catch with him, like every other father and son. I imagined taking my beautiful wife dancing. To say that Dr. Stoll's Immersion program transformed my life would be an understatement. As I've said, prior to meeting Dr. Stoll, I had spent close to twenty years struggling with all aspects of my health—facets that went far beyond just weight. Before attending his program, I had never had a doctor tell me I was in control of my health. I had always thought I was a victim of my genetics. I had considered my heritage to be the biggest influence on my physical state. My father had suffered from high blood pressure, so I would have high blood pressure, I had thought. I had also been told many,

many times that, as an African American, I would likely have high cholesterol and die early of heart disease or stroke. I had assumed my whole life, in a sense, had been predetermined. Immersion taught me otherwise.

Upon leaving the retreat and getting back to home life, I continued to follow the principles I had learned at immersion. Every day I would head to the gym and spend at least sixty minutes walking on a treadmill. Within three months, I had lost an additional seventy pounds and my doctor had taken me off all my medications. I was surprised by how quickly my body was responding to my new lifestyle. Everyone at the Whole Foods Market at which I worked took notice of the difference in me and threw their support behind me. It felt as though they were walking my journey alongside me.

At around the four-month mark of my new lifestyle, I was contacted by John Mackey of Whole Foods Market. I couldn't believe the cofounder of Whole Foods was reaching out to me, but evidently he had heard about my immersion experience and wanted to see how I was doing. When I told him of my weight loss, he congratulated me and asked if he could keep in touch. I was floored by his concern, and completely oblivious to the opportunities my immersion experience still held in store for me.

BRAND NEW

About six months after returning home from immersion, it became clear to me that I desperately needed to buy new clothing. I had lost over one hundred pounds. My body was changing. I had been forced to punch several new holes in my belts, which were now much too big for my waist. My pants and shirts had begun to swallow me up. Iris agreed that maybe it was time I went shopping. I had actually been avoiding making any wardrobe purchases, as I knew I was just getting started on my journey, but I decided to pick up a couple of pairs of jeans and a new belt to get me to my next milestone without looking silly.

Being a creature of habit, I jumped in my car and headed to my favorite clothing store. It was a "big and tall" store, of course. When I arrived, the manager, who knew me by name, asked me how I had been. He mentioned that I looked like I had lost weight, and asked me if I had been dieting. I laughed and told him I hadn't been dieting, per se, but had decided instead to make a lifestyle change. He asked me what I meant. I told him I no longer ate meat, dairy, or eggs. He said, "You're vegan?" I nodded my head, expecting a dubious look, but he just smiled and told me he was, too. We continued chatting as I searched for some new clothes.

I grabbed a pair of jeans I liked, and then made my way to the dressing rooms. I tried them on and immediately saw they were too baggy. I double-checked that I had taken a size forty-four. I had. I asked the manager if he had anything smaller, but he said he did not. He jokingly said he was going to be sad to lose me as a customer. After all, I had been shopping at his store for years. He suggested I go to the nearby mall and peruse the department stores. I couldn't remember the last time I had shopped for myself at a mall. What he said next caught me completely off guard. "You can buy clothes pretty much anywhere now," he said, hanging up the pants I had just tried on.

I was incredibly nervous as I drove my car across the huge parking lot surrounding the mall and found a spot right in front of one of the department stores. I walked inside and headed to the men's section, where I was greeted by a short middle-aged woman with dark hair and fair skin. She asked me if she could help me find anything. I told her what I needed, and then she asked me a question that any normal person would have been able to answer right away. She asked me what size pants I wore. At first I pretended I hadn't heard her as I followed her over to the area where all the jeans were. She turned and asked me again. Feeling a little embarrassed, I explained that I really didn't know what size I was. I shared the fact that I had recently lost a lot of weight. She grabbed a tape measure and asked me more about my story.

I told her all about my immersion experience and she asked me what size I was before the retreat. "Fifty-six-inch waist," I said. She gasped. Then she looked at me and said, "You now have a forty-inch waistline." I stood there in disbelief. As they had at my last day of immersion, tears of joy started rolling down my face. Before I knew it, the sales clerk was crying as well. She admitted how she wished her husband would lose some weight because it was starting to affect his health adversely. "Did you say your job paid to send you to this program?" she said. When I told her that was the case, she looked stunned. "Why would they do that?" she said. I smiled and told her that the company tries to improve the lives of the people that work for it. She chuckled and said she should pick up a job application for her husband on her way home.

The clerk pointed to a wall lined with jeans. I was in awe of the selection. There were more colors and styles than I had seen in a very long time. I wasn't even sure where to begin. After trying on several pairs, I selected two, as well as a new belt, and headed for the checkout line. The saleslady told me that if I had not mentioned my former obesity she would have never guessed it. I sincerely thanked her for all her help.

After paying for the clothes, I walked back to my car and called Iris. She asked how my shopping was going. I told her what had happened, but it did not surprise her. She said all the hard work I had been doing was really starting to pay off. It actually felt great not to hear any sort of astonishment in her voice. These changes were becoming my new normal.

MY SUPERHERO

In early spring, my former roommate, Michael, and I arranged to meet for dinner and a basketball game. We had not seen each other since the day we had left Florida. When I answered my doorbell, Michael looked at me and said, "Wow, Milan, you don't even look like the same person." I told him I was down about one hundred pounds, but that I still had a long way to go. He asked if I would be applying to go back to immersion as a reveal. I said I was certainly considering it. Michael said I definitely had to do it. He was positive I would be chosen. It was really nice to hear his enthusiasm. He really thought my story and results would motivate others.

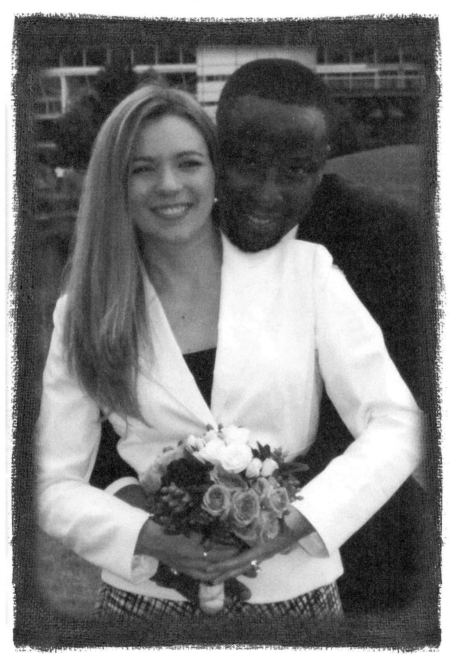

Milan and his biggest supporter, Iris.

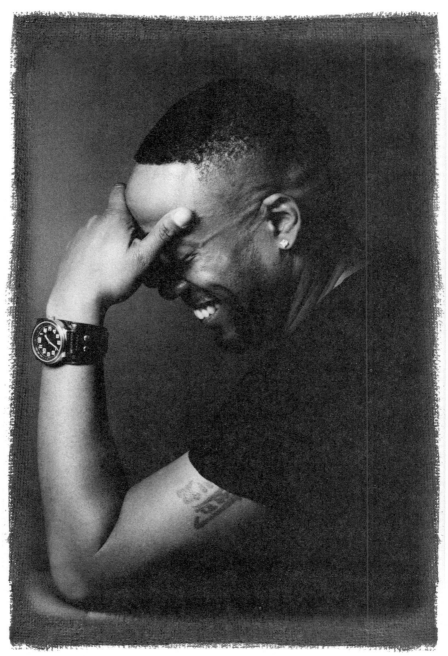

Milan taking a moment to appreciate his transformation.

In late May of 2014, I applied to be a reveal at the upcoming immersion and was accepted. I was down a total of one hundred and ten pounds with no desire to stop there. I found out that José, from my extended patio family at the retreat, would be the other reveal. He had also been morbidly obese before joining the program. Now he was well on his way to health, having lost over sixty pounds. It was hard to believe that immersion had helped us accomplish goals that had seemed virtually impossible to reach only six months prior.

By the time I reached the eighteen-month mark of my journey, I was down one hundred and seventy pounds and my entire life was different. I could fully engage myself in my son's interests. I could even pitch in as coach of his baseball, basketball, or football team when needed. Nigel and I had always had a strong bond between us, but now it was unbreakable. In fact, we became so close that he felt comfortable admitting to me how tough life with such an unhealthy father had been on him.

One day, as I was picking my son up from school, I happened to be wearing a Green Lantern T-shirt. My son's friends jokingly said I looked like a superhero now. Nigel seemed pretty excited by these comments. As we made our way to the car, Nigel said, "Could you wear your Green Lantern T-shirt the next time you pick me up?" I said I'd do my best, but probably wouldn't be able to keep it clean for every pick-up. Nigel got quiet. I asked him if he was all right. With tears in his eyes, he shared with me what things had been like for him when I was obese. He described how the kids would tease him whenever I'd pull up to his school. He said today was the first time they had said something nice.

I sat there listening to Nigel. When I asked him why he hadn't told me about any of this before, he said, "Dad, I didn't want to hurt your feelings." I realized Nigel had been protecting me for longer than I cared to admit. He was the superhero, not me. I told him none of it had been his fault. I also told him how sorry I was. My unhealthy lifestyle had caused him pain, and it crushed me to know it. I made sure Nigel knew he could talk to me about anything, no matter the subject matter. Then I kissed my son and told him I loved him.

ONLY HUMAN

As I write this, I have lost approximately two hundred and twenty-five pounds and taken more than twenty-five inches off my waistline. I have been able to discontinue all my prescription medications as well. There is not one part of my life that has not been affected by my decision to change my lifestyle. Moreover, one of the most rewarding aspects of my experience has been discovering that anyone can do what I have done. I am not special. In fact, I am one of the most ordinary people you could meet. I do not possess superhuman willpower, nor am I a trained chef. I have been successful simply because I have applied the principles of Dr. Stoll's Immersion program to my everyday life. If I can do it, I assure you, you can do it.

People sometimes ask me why I would want to reveal some of my most vulnerable moments with the world. The truth is that I would like everyone who still struggles as I did to know they have control over their own futures. By sharing my story, I hope others will understand they can change, too.

$\mathcal{D}$r. Stoll's Story

One of the greatest rewards of my professional life is the sight of a beaming smile on the face of an immersion attendee as he or she says, "I feel alive again!" It is incredibly satisfying to know that a person can be changed so dramatically in just one week thanks to solid scientific material and good, healthy meals. I cannot quite put into words the feeling I get from witnessing a program participant freed from the hopelessness of a seemingly inescapable situation, enlightened by information that shows a clear path forward, and empowered by a new understanding of the gift of choice and the reality of personal potential. There is nothing like seeing a person come alive again, full of energy, vitality, passion, and purpose.

The immersion program has provided the opportunity of reclaiming a healthy life to so many people, but it has transformed me just as powerfully. I, too, feel alive again. At one time in my medical career, I was physically and emotionally exhausted by the workload of a busy practice, frequently falling asleep on the couch before bed on Friday night and barely recovering over weekends, after which I would start the entire process again. Like most physicians, I went into medicine to help people, but I was struggling with the fact that I could not offer a real solution to the health problems that were profoundly affecting the quality of many of my patients' lives. It felt as though I was simply handing out Band-Aids all day.

Thankfully, an infusion of research on plant-based nutrition, stress and other emotional issues, and lifestyle interventions helped me see beyond my dissatisfaction and realize I could make a real difference in people's well-being. It rekindled hope in my profession of choice, and this hope truly caught fire as I began to see my patients' lives transformed by this information. As people shared with me how their symptoms had resolved after lifestyle changes, fresh energy filled the exam rooms of my practice I was able to discontinue medications for many of my patients, often saying, "It looks like I will be seeing you at the salad bar more frequently than I will in my office, because you don't really need to see me here so much anymore." I began to receive gifts from my patients, including bunches of kale, apples, fresh tomatoes, strawberries, and other delicious produce. Their gratitude was overwhelming. I loved practicing medicine in its purest form by regarding food and lifestyle as its foundation and restoring the health of people in need.

I have come to believe the solution to the global healthcare crisis is a grassroots movement of healthcare professionals rising up to lead their patients toward a lifestyle that sustains good health. Tens of thousands of people in the field have already embraced this philosophy, and more are doing so every day. It inspired me, in fact, to cofound a nonprofit organization called the Plantrician Project and a conference known as The International Plant Based Nutrition Healthcare Conference (www.PBNHC.com) to help educate other professionals on the scientific and medical research supporting the use of plant-based nutrition in healthcare.

I was given a priceless gift when Whole Foods asked me to host a seven-day health retreat, and I will forever be grateful for John Mackey's support and encouragement. The retreat continues to be an invaluable opportunity for me to learn more about the process of changing lifestyle habits, the power of food, and the strength of a unified team. The immersion program afforded me the unexpected and unique ability to include my family in my work. It is utterly heartwarming to me that each member of my family now actively participates in the week, sharing in the labor and joy of helping others.

My children have benefited immensely from the time they have spent at immersion. They have met people from around the world and every walk of life, and have learned that we are all inherently the same. Before every retreat, we always take time as a family to pray for the people that will be in attendance and wonder aloud about the amazing stories that might develop during the week. Each immersion experience becomes a priceless and treasured family memory that we know we will discuss with each other for the rest of our lives.

THE CATALYST

I have always believed in the ability of every individual to change, but the process sometimes requires a catalyst—a person or team that is ready and willing to offer a helping hand. The immersion program has been this helping hand to so many who were in real need of it, who simply didn't know where to begin. Whole Foods has created a platform that gives every team member, independent of position, the opportunity to find solutions to their health challenges.

The process of working with people as they adjust core foundations of their lives such as diet and behavior has taught me many life lessons. For example, I now see that food is intimately connected to every aspect of a person's life, and that the process of change uncovers layers of emotion, which sometimes include pain from the past. For some, success is hindered by an emotional burden, and the key step forward is to obtain freedom from this emotional pain. When I started this immersion program, I never expected to explore so deeply the emotional component of eating, but I have come to believe it is critical to do so in order to find true health. Deep-seated emotions can cause a person to turn to eating as a method of regaining a sense of control or comfort, most often unconsciously. With this in mind, I frequently refer immersionists to other professionals who might help them achieve permanent emotional healing as they work toward improving their physical health.

The countless hours I have spent thinking about food have opened my eyes to the connectedness of the world and the fact that decisions never affect just one aspect of life. The simple food choice you make at a grocery store is part of a chain of events that begins by caring for the soil and ends with the disposal of any refuse left behind after a meal. This chain includes growing the food, harvesting it, shipping it, consuming it, and experiencing the ways in which it affects your health. The decisions you make today create not only your future but also the future of the larger world. One bite at a time, you impact, whether positively or negatively, not only your health but also the health of the environment.

Stewardship is the responsible management of an item or task with which one has been entrusted. In regard to food, that item is the planet Earth. Stewardship is a foundational principle of my life and one that I teach my children. We are all stewards of the land, as the health of the soil, and thus the health of plants and the people who eat them, will be passed on as an inheritance to our children. As stewards, I believe we should base our decisions not on immediate gratification but rather on a vision of tomorrow.

Many people, however, consider merely the present moment when deciding what to eat. No one has taught them how to think about food differently, so they opt for that with which they are familiar, which may not be the best choice in terms of health or the environment. My friendships with organic farmers have afforded me a new understanding of food. I now know how important it is to be a conscious consumer. I recognize the link between food, the environment, and the future of generations to come. I am fortunate that my immersion program allows me to witness people taking their first steps toward acknowledging this idea as well.

THE CHRYSALIS

The immersion experience and this book are tools to help people achieve renewed health and a new mindset. They are meant to set people free from old habits that have been holding them back from attaining full, happy lives. It is my life's passion to see people transformed by the ideas contained in these pages. Although it may sound like a cliché, I truly believe the essence of this program is best depicted by the way in which a caterpillar becomes a butterfly.

Prior to undergoing its metamorphosis into a butterfly, a caterpillar eats all the food required to fuel this transformation. Filled to capacity, the caterpillar finds a suitable place, preferably out of the way of danger, and then forms a chrysalis in preparation for this amazing change. Inside the chrysalis, a remarkable process begins. The caterpillar releases enzymes that dissolve all its tissues, digesting itself, in a way. All that remains in the chrysalis is a protein-rich soup and several sets of tiny cells. These sets are known as imaginal discs, which are very similar to embryonic cells. These discs generally lie dormant in a caterpillar until the protein-rich fluid in the chrysalis helps them form the new adult structures that will make up the butterfly—eyes, legs, antennae, wings, etc. Imaginal discs actually overcome the immune system of a caterpillar, which sees them as foreign bodies, to create a butterfly. Once it has fully matured, the butterfly breaks through the chrysalis, spreads its wings, and eventually leaves its old shell behind.

As the caterpillar must consume large amounts of food in order to have the energy necessary to transform itself, immersionists must take in as much information as they can to prepare themselves to undergo a big change. This information fuels transformation. As the caterpillar looks for an out-of-the-way spot to turn into a butterfly, immersionists should pull back from the business of life when attempting to shed old habits and adopt a new lifestyle.

Time and time again, I've seen immersion attendees bring with them untapped potential that has been dormant throughout their lives, much like the caterpillar's imaginal discs. Immersion acts as the beginning of the process of change for participants. It breaks down the walls and mindsets that have held them back, igniting the potential inside each of them and creating completely new lives.

Once participants leave the retreat, real change permeates every area of their lives and they welcome and embrace their new states with acceptance and gratitude. They go on to spend several months working through the daily steps of their new habits and releasing old mindsets. Before long, the lifestyle demonstrated at immersion has become second nature. They've changed for good. And what is even more exciting is that this type of transformation tends to attract others, who then learn the message of this book and change themselves, creating a powerful chain reaction. Certainly this has been the case with Milan, who seems to inspire everyone who meets him.

Today, right now, you possess the ability to alter the course of your life for the better by making a positive choice for your health. You may then build upon that choice by making more and more positive decisions each day, as though you are taking steps in the direction of a better place. Instead of stopping at your destination, however, you will simply continue moving ahead. Don't be overwhelmed by the idea of overhauling your entire life; just focus on the moment. Understanding the science of nutrition and human biology is part of the process of achieving lasting health, but it should not overshadow your focus on the simplicity and power of your daily decisions. At the end of the day, the answer you've been looking for is easy to find: Decide to eat well, move more, sleep more, and stress less.

You are not stuck in the life you are leading. You now have the information you require to make *The Change*. Even though it seems the escalator of life has broken down, all you need to do is take it one step at a time and you'll soon find yourself reaching a new level you never thought you'd see, and experiencing a sense of freedom you never thought possible.

References

Getting on Board

1. Ayyad, C., and T. Andersen. "Long-term efficacy of dietary treatment of obesity: a systematic review of studies published between 1931 and 1999." *Obes Rev* 1.2 (2000): 113–119.

2. Barnard R.J., Massey M.R., Cherny S., O'Brien L.T., and N. Pritikin. "Long-term use of a high-complex-carbohydrate, high-fiber, low-fat diet and exercise in the treatment of NIDDM patients." *Diabetes Care* 6.3 (1983): 268–273.

3. McDougall, John, and Laurie E. Thomas. "Effects of 7 days on an ad libitum low-fat vegan diet: the McDougall Program cohort." *Nutrition Journal* 13.1 (2014): 1–7.

Day Two

1. Emmons, Robert A., and Charles M. Shelton. "Gratitude and the science of positive psychology." *Handbook of Positive Psychology* 18 (2002): 459–471.

2. Wood, Alex M., Froh, Jeffrey J., and Adam W.A. Geraghty. "Gratitude and well-being: A review and theoretical integration." *Clin Psychol Rev* 30.7 (2010): 890–905.

3. Mills, Paul J., et al. "The role of gratitude in spiritual well-being in asymptomatic heart failure patients." *Spiritual Clin Pract* 2.1 (2015): 5–17.

4. O'Connor, C. M., Jiang, W., Kuchibhatla, M., Silva, S.G., Cuffe, M. S., and D.D. Callwood. "Safety and efficacy of sertraline for depression in patients with heart failure: Results of the SADHART-CHF (Sertraline Against Depression and Heart Disease in Chronic Heart Failure) trial." *J Am Coll Cardiol* 56.9 (2010): 692–699.

Day Three

1. Li, Jie, et al. "Improvement in chewing activity reduces energy intake in one meal and modulates plasma gut hormone concentrations in obese and lean young Chinese men." *Am J Clin Nutr* 94.3 (2011): 709–716.

2. Kokkinos, Alexander, et al. "Eating slowly increases the postprandial response of the anorexigenic gut hormones, peptide YY and glucagon-like peptide-1." *J Clin Endocrinol Metab* 95.1 (2010): 333–337.

3. Crujeiras, Ana B., et al. "Weight regain after a diet-induced loss is predicted by higher baseline leptin and lower ghrelin plasma levels." *J Clin Endocrinol Metab* 95.11 (2010): 5037–5044.

4. Klok, M. D., Jakobsdottir, S., and M. L. Drent. "The role of leptin and ghrelin in the regulation of food intake and body weight in humans: a review." *Obes Rev* 8.1 (2007): 21–34.

5. Weigle, D.S., Cummings, D.E., Newby, P.D., Breen, P.A., Frayo, R.S., Matthys, C.C., Callahan, H.S., and J.Q. Purnell. "Roles of leptin and ghrelin in the loss of body weight caused by a low fat, high carbohydrate diet." *J Clin Endocrinol Metab* 88.4 (2003): 1577–1586.

6. Gearhardt, A.N., Grilo, C.M., DiLeone, R.L., Brownell, K.D., and M.N. Potenza. "Can food be addictive? Public health and policy implications." *Addiction* 106.7 (2011): 1208–1212.

7. Volkow, Nora D., et al. "Low dopamine striatal D2 receptors are associated with prefrontal metabolism in obese subjects: possible contributing factors." *Neuroimage* 42.4 (2008): 1537–1543.

8. Wang, Gene-Jack, et al. "Exposure to appetitive food stimuli markedly activates the human brain." *Neuroimage* 21.4 (2004): 1790–1797.

9. Pelchat, Marcia Levin, et al. "Images of desire: food-craving activation during fMRI." *Neuroimage* 23.4 (2004): 1486–1493.

10. Avena, N.M., Rada, P., and B.G. Hoebel. "Evidence for sugar addiction: Behavioral and neurochemical effects of intermittent, excessive sugar intake." *Neurosci Biobehav Rev* 32.1 (2008): 20–39.

11. Ahmed, Serge H., Guillem, K., and Youna Vandaele. "Sugar addiction: pushing the drug-sugar analogy to the limit." *Curr Opin Clin Nutr Metab Care* 16.4 (2013): 434–439.

12. Drewnoski, A., Krahn, D.D., Demitrack, M.A., Nairn, K., and B.A. Gosnell. "Taste responses and preferences for sweet high-fat foods: evidence for opioid involvement." *Physiol Behav* 51.2 (1992): 371–379.

13. Lenoir, Magalie, et al. "Intense sweetness surpasses cocaine reward." *PLoS ONE* 2.8 (2007): e698.

14. Heng, H.Y., and H.R. Berthoud. "Neural systems controlling the drive to eat: mind versus metabolism." *Physiology* 23.2 (2008): 75.

15. Kurek, M., Przybilla, B., Hermann, K., and J. Ring. "A naturally occurring opioid peptide from cow's milk, beta-casomorphine-7, is a direct histamine releaser in man." *Int Arch Allergy Immunol* 97.2 (1992): 115–120.

16. Parker, M. Rockwell, et al. "Expression and nuclear translocation of glucocorticoid receptors in type 2 taste receptor cells." *Neuroscience Letters* 571 (2014): 72–77.

17. Neylan, Thomas C. "Hans Selye and the Field of Stress Research." *J Neuropsych Clin N* 10.2 (1998): 230.

18. Kiecolt-Glaser, J.K., McGuire, L., Robles, T.F., and Ronald Glaser. "Psychoneuroimmunology: Psychological influences on immune function and health." *J Consult Clin Psychol* 70.3 (2002): 537–547.

Day Four

1. Conover, Chris. "The Cost of Health Care: 1958 vs. 2012." Forbes. December 12, 2012. Accessed February 25, 2016. http://www.forbes.com/sites/chrisconover/2012/12/22/the-cost-of-health-care-1958-vs-2012/#7bc3537d590f.

2. Drewnowski, A. "The cost of US foods as related to their nutritive value." *Am J Clin Nutr* 92.5 (2010): 1181–1188.

3. Bernstein, Adam M., et al. "Relation of food cost to healthfulness of diet among US women." *Am J Clin Nutr* 92.5 (2010): 1197–1203.

4. Coyne, Mark S., et al. "Soil microorganisms contribute to plant nutrition and root health." *Better Crops with Plant Food* 99.1 (2015): 18–20.

5. Prasad, R., Kumar, M., and Ajit Varma. "Role of PGPR in Soil Fertility and Plant Health." *Plant-Growth-Promoting Rhizobacteria (PGPR) and Medicinal Plants.* Springer International Publishing, 2015: 247–260.

6. Davis, Donald R. "Declining fruit and vegetable nutrient composition: What is the evidence?" *HortScience* 44.1 (2009): 15–19.

7. Mayer, Anne-Marie. "Historical changes in the mineral content of fruits and vegetables." *British Food Journal* 99.6 (1997): 207–211.

8. Hung, H.C., Joshipura, K.J., Jiang, R., et al. "Fruit and vegetable intake and risk of major chronic disease." *J Natl Cancer Inst* 96.21 (2004): 1577–1584.

9. World Cancer Research Fund/American Institute for Cancer Research. *Food, Nutrition, Physical Activity, and the Prevention of Cancer: a Global Perspective.* Washington, D.C.: American Institute for Cancer Research, 2007.

10. Slavin, J.L., and B. Lloyd. "Health benefits of fruits and vegetables." *Adv Nutr* 3.4 (2012): 506–516.

11. Subramoniam, Appian, et al. "Chlorophyll Revisited: Anti-inflammatory Activities of Chlorophyll a and Inhibition of Expression of TNF-α Gene by the Same." *Inflammation* 35.3 (2012): 959–966.

12. Lin, Kuan-Hung, et al. "Chlorophyll-related compounds inhibit cell adhesion and inflammation in human aortic cells." *J Med Food* 16.10 (2013): 886–898.

13. Singh, Karnail, et al. "Effect of wheat grass tablets on the frequency of blood transfusions in Thalassemia Major." *Indian J Pediatr* 77.1 (2010): 90–91.

14. Marwaha, R. K., et al. "Wheat grass juice reduces transfusion requirement in patients with thalassemia major: a pilot study." *Indian J Pediatr* 41.7 (2004): 716–720.

15. Liu, Rui Hai. "Health benefits of fruit and vegetables are from additive and synergistic combinations of phytochemicals." *Am J Clin Nutr* 78.3 (2003): 517S–520S.

16. Liu, Rui Hai. "Potential synergy of phytochemicals in cancer prevention: mechanism of action." *J Nutr* 134.12 (2004): 3479S–3485S.

17. Park, Madison. "Twinkie diet helps nutrition professor lose 27 pounds." CNN. November 8, 2010. Accessed December 12, 2012. http://www.cnn.com/2010/ HEALTH/11/08/twinkie.diet.professor/

18. Schoeller, Dale A. "Limitations in the assessment of dietary energy intake by self-report." *Metabolism* 44.2.2 (1995): 18–22.

19. Lichtman, Steven W., et al. "Discrepancy between self-reported and actual caloric intake and exercise in obese subjects." *N Engl J Med* 327.27 (1992): 1893–1898.

20. Duncan, Karen H., Bacon, Jane A., and Roland L. Weinsier. "The effects of high and low energy density diets on satiety, energy intake, and eating time of obese and nonobese subjects." *Am J Clin Nutr* 37.5 (1983): 763–767.

21. Shintani, Terry T., et al. "Obesity and cardiovascular risk intervention through the ad libitum feeding of traditional Hawaiian diet." *Am J Clin Nutr* 53.6 (1991): 1647S–1651S.

22. Vad Andersen, B., and Grethe Hyldig. "Food satisfaction: Integrating feelings before, during and after food intake." *Food Quality and Preference* 43 (2015): 126–134.

23. Liu, Rui Hai. "Health benefits of fruit and vegetables are from additive and synergistic combinations of phytochemicals." *Am J Clin Nutr* 78.3 (2003): 517S–520S.

24. Berenson, Gerald S., et al. "Atherosclerosis of the aorta and coronary arteries and cardiovascular risk factors in persons aged 6 to 30 years and

studied at necropsy (The Bogalusa Heart Study)." *Am J Cardiol* 70.9 (1992): 851–858.

25. Tuzcu, E. Murat, et al. "High prevalence of coronary atherosclerosis in asymptomatic teenagers and young adults: evidence from intravascular ultrasound." *Circulation* 103.22 (2001): 2705–2710.

26. Joseph, A., Ackerman, D., Talley, J., Johnstone, J., and J. Kupersmith. "Manifestations of coronary atherosclerosis in young trauma victims–an autopsy study." *J Am Coll Cardiol* 22.2 (1993): 459–467.

27. Shirani, J., Yousefi, J., and William C. Roberts. "Major cardiac findings at necropsy in 366 American octogenarians." *Am J Cardiol* 75.2 (1995): 151–156.

Day Five

1. Ayyad, C., and T. Andersen. "Long-term efficacy of dietary treatment of obesity: a systematic review of studies published between 1931 and 1999." *Obes Rev* 1.2 (2000): 113–119.

2. Serruys, P.W., Luijten, H.E., Beatt, K.J., et al. "Incidence of restenosis after successful coronary angioplasty: a time-related phenomenon: a quantitative angiographic study in 342 consecutive patients at 1, 2, 3, and 4 months." *Circulation* 77.2 (1988): 361–371.

3. Simoons, M. L. "Reocclusion/restenosis after coronary artery bypass surgery, percutaneous transluminal coronary angioplasty and thrombolysis." *Z Kardiol* 78.3 (1989): 35–41.

4. Johnson, Ian T. "Glucosinolates: bioavailability and importance to health." *Int J Vitam Nutr Res* 72.1 (2002): 26–31.

5. Tang, Li, et al. "Consumption of raw cruciferous vegetables is inversely associated with bladder cancer risk." *Cancer Epidemiol Biomarkers Prev* 17.4 (2008): 938–944.

6. Kopic, S., and John P. Geibel. "Gastric acid, calcium absorption, and their impact on bone health." *Physiol Rev* 93.1 (2013): 189–268.

7. Famularo, G., Gasbarrone, L., and Giovanni Minisola. "Hypomagnesemia and proton-pump inhibitors." *Expert Opinion on Drug Safety* 12.5 (2013): 709–716.

8. Fasano, A. "Leaky gut and autoimmune diseases." *Clin Rev Allergy Immunol* 42.1 (2012): 71–78.

9. Widlansky, Michael E., et al. "The clinical implications of endothelial dysfunction." *Journal of the American College of Cardiology* 42.7 (2003): 1149–1160.

10. Lopez-Garcia, Esther, et al. "Consumption of trans fatty acids is related to plasma biomarkers of inflammation and endothelial dysfunction." *J Nutr* 135.3 (2005): 562–566.

11. Institute of Medicine of the National Academies. *Dietary Reference Intakes for Energy, Carbohydrate, Fiber, Fat, Fatty Acids, Cholesterol, Protein, and Amino Acids.* Washington, D.C.: National Academies Press, 2003.

12. Lopez-Garcia, Esther, et al. "Major dietary patterns are related to plasma concentrations of markers of inflammation and endothelial dysfunction." *Am J Clin Nutr* 80.4 (2004): 1029–1035.

13. Lekakis, John, et al. "Polyphenols compounds from red grapes acutely improve endothelial function in patients with coronary heart disease." *Eur J Cardiovasc Prev Rehabil* 12.6 (2005): 596–600.

14. Tuso, P., Stoll, S.R., and William W. Li. "A plant-based diet, atherogenesis, and coronary artery disease prevention." *Perm J* 19.1 (2015): 62–67.

15. Ornish, Dean, et al. "Can lifestyle changes reverse coronary heart disease? The Lifestyle Heart Trial." *Lancet* 336.8708 (1990): 129–133.

16. Gould, K. Lance, et al. "Changes in myocardial perfusion abnormalities by positron emission tomography after long-term, intense risk factor modification." *JAMA* 274.11 (1995): 894–901.

17. Ornish, Dean, et al. "Intensive lifestyle changes for reversal of coronary heart disease." *JAMA* 280.23 (1998): 2001–2007.

18. Esselstyn, Caldwell B. "Resolving the Coronary Artery Disease Epidemic Through Plant-Based Nutrition." *Preventive cardiology* 4.4 (2001): 171–177.

19. Mesquita, D.N., Barbieri, M.A., Goldani, H.A., Cardoso, V.C., Goldani, M.Z., Kac, G., et al. "Cesarean Section Is Associated with Increased Peripheral and Central Adiposity in Young Adulthood: Cohort Study." *PLoS One* 8.6 (2013): e66827.

20. Jost, Ted, et al. "Vertical mother–neonate transfer of maternal gut bacteria via breastfeeding." *Environ Microbiol* 16.9 (2014): 2891–2904.

21. Turnbaugh, Peter J., et al. "The effect of diet on the human gut microbiome: a metagenomic analysis in humanized gnotobiotic mice." *Sci Transl Med* 1.6 (2009): 6ra14–6ra14.

22. David, Lawrence A., et al. "Diet rapidly and reproducibly alters the human gut microbiome." *Nature* 505 (2014): 559–563.

23. Tang, W. H., and Stanley L. Hazen. "The contributory role of gut microbiota in cardiovascular disease." *J Clin Invest* 124.10 (2014): 4204–4211.

24. Koeth, Robert A., et al. "Intestinal microbiota metabolism of L-carnitine, a nutrient in red meat, promotes atherosclerosis." *Nature Medicine* 19 (2013): 576–585.

25. Xu, R., QuanQiu ,W., and Li Li. "A genome-wide systems analysis reveals

strong link between colorectal cancer and trimethylamine N-oxide (TMAO), a gut microbial metabolite of dietary meat and fat." *BMC Genomics* 16.Suppl 7 (2015): S4.

26. Tang, W.H., Wang, Z., Levison, B.S., et al. "Intestinal Microbial Metabolism of Phosphatidylcholine and Cardiovascular Risk." *N Engl J Med* 368.17 (2013): 1575–1584.

27. Painter, Neil S., and Denis P. Burkitt. "Diverticular disease of the colon: a deficiency disease of Western civilization." *Br Med J* 2 (1971): 450–454.

28. Spiller, R. C. "Changing views on diverticular disease: impact of aging, obesity, diet, and microbiota." *Neurogastroenterol Motil* 27.3 (2015): 305–312.

29. Amre, D.K., D'Souza, S., Morgan, K., et al. "Imbalances in dietary consumption of fatty acids, vegetables, and fruits are associated with risk for Crohn's disease in children." *Am J Gastroenterol* 102.9 (2007): 2016–2025.

30. Wu, G.D., Chen, J., Hoffmann, C., et al. "Linking long-term dietary patterns with gut microbial enterotypes." *Science* 334.6052 (2011):105–108.

31. Nanda, R., et al. "Food intolerance and the irritable bowel syndrome." *Gut* 30.8 (1989): 1099–1104.

32. Bai, S.K., Lee, S.J., Na, H.J., et al . "beta-Carotene inhibits inflammatory gene expression in lipopolysaccharide-stimulated macrophages by suppressing redox-based NF-kappaB activation." *Ex Mol Med* 37.4 (2005): 323–334.

33. Nagy-Szakal, D., Hollister, E.B., Luna, R.A., et al. "Cellulose supplementation early in life ameliorates colitis in adult mice." *PLoS One* 8.2 (2103): e56685.

34. Pan, An, et al. "Red meat consumption and mortality: results from 2 prospective cohort studies." *Archives of internal medicine* 172.7 (2012): 555-563.

35. Sinha, Rashmi, et al. "Meat intake and mortality: a prospective study of over half a million people." *Arch Intern Med* 169.6 (2009): 562–571.

36. Bastide, Nadia M., Fabrice, H.F. Pierre, and Denis E. Corpet. "Heme iron from meat and risk of colorectal cancer: a meta-analysis and a review of the mechanisms involved." *Cancer Prev Res* 4.2 (2011): 177–184.

37. Ascherio, Alberto, et al. "Dietary iron intake and risk of coronary disease among men." *Circulation* 89.3 (1994): 969–974.

38. Yang, Wei, et al. "Is heme iron intake associated with risk of coronary heart disease? A meta-analysis of prospective studies." *Eur J Nutr* 53.2 (2014): 395–400.

39. Brown, K., DeCoffe, D., Molcan, E., and D.L. Gibson. "Diet-Induced Dysbiosis of the Intestinal Microbiota and the Effects on Immunity and Disease." *Nutrients* 4.8 (2012): 1095–1119.

40. Padler-Karavani, Vered, et al. "Diversity in specificity, abundance, and composition of anti-Neu5Gc antibodies in normal humans: potential implications for disease." *Glycobiology* 18.10 (2008): 818–830.

41. Fontana L, et al. "Long-term effects of calorie or protein restriction on serum IGF-1 and IGFBP-3 concentration in humans." *Aging Cell* 7.5 (2008): 681–687.

42. Murphy, Neil, et al. "Dietary fibre intake and risks of cancers of the colon and rectum in the European prospective investigation into cancer and nutrition (EPIC)." *PLoS One* 7.6 (2012): e39361.

43. Liu, Guiyuan, et al. "Inositol hexaphosphate suppresses growth and induces apoptosis in HT-29 colorectal cancer cells in culture: PI3K/Akt pathway as a potential target." *Int J Clin Exp Path* 8.2 (2015): 1402–1410.

44. Wang, Min, et al. "Effects of phytochemicals sulforaphane on uridine diphosphate-glucuronosyltransferase expression as well as cell-cycle arrest and apoptosis in human colon cancer Caco-2 cells." *Chin J Physiol* 55.2 (2012): 134–144.

45. Madka, V., and Chinthalapally V. Rao. "Anti-inflammatory phytochemicals for chemoprevention of colon cancer." *Curr Cancer Drug Targets* 13.5 (2013): 542–557.

46. Madka, V., and Chinthalapally V. Rao. "Anti-inflammatory phytochemicals for chemoprevention of colon cancer." *Curr Cancer Drug Targets* 13.5 (2013): 542–557.

Day Six

1. Khaw, Kay-Tee, et al. "Association of hemoglobin A1c with cardiovascular disease and mortality in adults: the European prospective investigation into cancer in Norfolk." *Ann Intern Med* 141.6 (2004): 413–420.

2. Selvin, E., Coresh, J., Golden, S.H., Brancati, F.L., Folsom, A.R., and M.W. Steffes. "Glycemic control and coronary heart disease risk in persons with and without diabetes: the atherosclerosis risk in communities study." *Arch Intern Med* 165.16 (2005): 1910–1916.

3. "National Diabetes Statistics Report, 2014." CDC. Accessed February 18, 2016. http://www.cdc.gov/diabetes/pubs/statsreport14/national-diabetes-report-web.pdf

4. *IDF Diabetes Atlas, Sixth Edition.* IDF. Accessed February 18, 2016. https://www .idf.org/sites/default/files/EN_6E_Atlas_Full_0.pdf

5. Sweeney, J. Shirley. "Dietary factors that influence the dextrose tolerance test: a preliminary study." *Arch Int Med* 40.6 (1927): 818–830.

6. Perseghin, Gianluca, et al. "Intramyocellular triglyceride content is a determinant of in vivo insulin resistance in humans: a 1H-13C nuclear magnetic resonance spectroscopy assessment in offspring of type 2 diabetic parents." *Diabetes* 48.8 (1999): 1600–1606.

7. Boden, Guenther, et al. "Effects of acute changes of plasma free fatty acids on intramyocellular fat content and insulin resistance in healthy subjects." *Diabetes* 50.7 (2001): 1612–1617.

8. Boden, G., and G. I. Shulman. "Free fatty acids in obesity and type 2 diabetes: defining their role in the development of insulin resistance and β-cell dysfunction." *Eur J Clin Invest* 32.s3 (2002): 14–23.

9. El-Assaad, Wissal, et al. "Saturated fatty acids synergize with elevated glucose to cause pancreatic β-cell death." *Endocrinology* 144.9 (2003): 4154–4163.

10. Luchsinger, José A., and Deborah R. Gustafson. "Adiposity, type 2 diabetes and Alzheimer's disease." *J Alzheimer's Dis* 16.4 (2009): 693–704.

11. Cnop, M., et al. "Low density lipoprotein can cause death of islet beta-cells by its cellular uptake and oxidative modification." *Endocrinology* 143.9 (2002): 3449–3453.

12. Tripathy, Devjit, et al. "Elevation of free fatty acids induces inflammation and impairs vascular reactivity in healthy subjects." *Diabetes* 52.12 (2003): 2882–2887.

13. Fraser, Gary E. "Vegetarian diets: what do we know of their effects on common chronic diseases?" *Am J Clin Nutr* 89.5 (2009): 1607S–1612S.

14. Goff, Louise M., et al. "Veganism and its relationship with insulin resistance and intramyocellular lipid." *Eur J Clin Nutr* 59.2 (2005): 291–298.

15. Tonstad, S., et al. "Vegetarian diets and incidence of diabetes in the Adventist Health Study-2." *Nutr Metab Cardiovasc Dis* 23.4 (2013): 292–299.

16. Kahleova, H., Hrachovinova, T., Hill, M., and T. Pelikanova. "Vegetarian diet in type 2 diabetes–improvement in quality of life, mood and eating behavior: A randomized, open, parallel, controlled trial." *Diabetic Medicine* 30 (2013): 127–129.

17. Anderson, James W., and Kyleen Ward. "High-carbohydrate, high-fiber diets for insulin-treated men with diabetes mellitus." *Am J Clin Nutr* 32.11 (1979): 2312–2321.

18. Barnard, R. James, et al. "Response of non-insulin-dependent diabetic patients to an intensive program of diet and exercise." *Diabetes Care* 5.4 (1982): 370–374.

19. Barnard, Neal D., et al. "A low-fat vegan diet improves glycemic control and cardiovascular risk factors in a randomized clinical trial in individuals with type 2 diabetes." *Diabetes Care* 29.8 (2006): 1777–1783.

20. Crane, Milton G., and Clyde Sample. "Regression of diabetic neuropathy with total vegetarian (vegan) diet." *J Nutr Med* 4.4 (1994): 431–439.

21. Kempner, W., Peschel, R.L., and C. Schlayer. "Effect of rice diet on diabetes mellitus associated with vascular disease." *Postgrad Med* 24.4 (1958): 359–371.

22. Roseboom, T., de Rooij, S., and R. Painter. "The Dutch famine and its long-term consequences for adult health." *Early Hum Dev* 82.8 (2006):485–491.

23. Kaati, G., et al. "Transgenerational response to nutrition, early life circumstances and longevity." *Eur J Hum Genet* 15.7 (2007): 784–790.

24. Jirtle, Randy L., and Michael K. Skinner. "Environmental epigenomics and disease susceptibility." *Nature Reviews Genetics* 8.4 (2007): 253–262.

25. Pasman, W. J., et al. "Nutrigenomics approach elucidates health-promoting effects of high vegetable intake in lean and obese men." *Genes Nutr* 8.5 (2013): 507–521.

26. Junien, Claudine. "Impact of diets and nutrients/drugs on early epigenetic programming." *J Inherit Metab Dis* 29.2–3 (2006): 359–365.

27. Fraser, Gary E. *Diet, Life Expectancy, and Chronic Disease: Studies of Seventh-Day Adventists and Other Vegetarians.* New York: Oxford University Press, 2003.

28. Singh, Pramil N., and Gary E. Fraser. "Dietary risk factors for colon cancer in a low-risk population." *Am J Epidemiol* 148.8 (1998): 761–774.

29. Ford, Earl S., et al. "Healthy living is the best revenge: findings from the European Prospective Investigation into Cancer and Nutrition-Potsdam study." *Arch Intern Med* 169.15 (2009): 1355–1362.

30. Folkman J. "Angiogenesis in cancer, vascular, rheumatoid and other disease." *Nat Med* 1 (1995): 27–31.

31. Elahy, Mina, et al. "Nicotine Attenuates Disruption of Blood–Brain Barrier Induced by Saturated-Fat Feeding in Wild-Type Mice." *Nicotine Tob Res* 17.12 (2015): 1436–1441.

32. Valenzuela, John P., et al. "Abstract W P388: High Fat and High Glucose Synergistically Impair Brain Microvascular Endothelial Cell Survival and Angiogenic Potential after Hypoxia." *Stroke* 46.Suppl 1 (2015): AWP388–AWP388.

33. Xie, Huixu, et al. "Chronic stress promotes oral cancer growth and angiogenesis with increased circulating catecholamine and glucocorticoid levels in a mouse model." *Oral Oncol* 51.11 (2015): 991–997.

34. Sponder, Michael, et al. "Physical inactivity increases endostatin and osteopontin in patients with coronary artery disease." *Heart and Vessels* (December 11, 2015): 1–6.

35. Albini, Adriana, et al. "Cancer prevention by targeting angiogenesis." *Nat Rev Clin Oncol* 9.9 (2012): 498–509.

36. Tan, Wen-fu, et al. "Quercetin, a dietary-derived flavonoid, possesses antiangiogenic potential." *Eur J Pharmacol* 459.2–3 (2003): 255–262.

37. Kasiotis, Konstantinos M., et al. "Resveratrol and related stilbenes: their anti-aging and anti-angiogenic properties." *Food Chem Toxicol* 61 (2013): 112–120.

38. Miyazawa, T., Kiyotaka, N., and Phumon Sookwong. "Health benefits of vitamin E in grains, cereals and green vegetables." *Trends in Food Science & Technology* 22.12 (2011): 651–654.

39. Antoni, Michael H., et al. "The influence of bio-behavioural factors on tumour biology: pathways and mechanisms." *Nat Rev Cancer* 6.3 (2006): 240–248.

40. Thaker, Premal H., et al. "Chronic stress promotes tumor growth and angiogenesis in a mouse model of ovarian carcinoma." *Nat Med* 12.8 (2006): 939–944.

41. Jones, Lee W., et al. "Effect of aerobic exercise on tumor physiology in an animal model of human breast cancer." *J Appl Physiol* 108.2 (2010): 343–348.

42. *Global Cancer Facts & Figures, 2nd Edition.* Atlanta: American Cancer Society, 2011.

Day Seven

1. Weaver, C.M., and K.L. Plawecki. "Dietary calcium: adequacy of a vegetarian diet." *Am J Clin Nutr* 59.5 (1994): 1238S–1241S.

2. Appleby, P., Roddam, A., Allen, N., and T. Key. "Comparative fracture risk in vegetarians and nonvegetarians in EPIC-Oxford." *Eur J Clin Nutr* 61.12 (2007): 1400–1406.

About the Authors

Milan Ross was born and raised in Saint Louis, Missouri, and graduated from Central Visual and Performing Arts High School with a passion for the arts. After pursuing a career in the music industry and getting married, his family was faced with a health crisis, which required him to find a job that provided health insurance to cover mounting medical bills. In 2012, Milan walked away from his career in music and took a position with Whole Foods Market. This fateful decision changed not only Milan's life but also the life of each member of his family.

As an overweight individual, Milan was intrigued by the health retreat offered by Whole Foods to its employees in need. He soon applied and was accepted. After attending Dr. Stoll's Immersion program in 2013, Milan lost over two hundred and twenty-five pounds. The story of his dramatic transformation broke nationally on the cover of *Vegan Lifestyle Magazine.* It has since been featured in several national magazines and highlighted in the feature-length documentary film *Eating You Alive.* In addition, Milan has developed his own organic health food line, Full Flavor Vegan (www.fullflavorvegan.com).

Today, through his many speaking engagements across the United States, Milan has made it his life's mission to help people attain optimal health and change their lives. Milan lives with his wife and son in Highlands Ranch, Colorado, where they are actively involved in serving their church and community.

Scott Stoll, MD, received his medical degree from the University of Colorado. He is board certified by the American Board of Physical Medicine and Rehabilitation and specializes in regenerative medicine, utilizing natural treatments, diet, and lifestyle to aid the body in healing chronic disease and injuries.

Prior to receiving his MD, he was a member of the 1994 US Olympic Bobsled team, and he currently serves as a physician for USA Bobsled & Skeleton. He is also cofounder of the Plantrician Project and the International Plant-Based Nutrition Healthcare Conference; has served as a member of the Whole Foods scientific and medical advisory board; is athletic team physician for Lehigh University; and is department chairman of Physical Medicine and Rehabilitation at Coordinated Health.

Beyond conducting his popular "Dr. Stoll's Immersion" program several times a year, Dr. Stoll is the author of *Alive! A Physician's Biblical & Scientific Guide to Nutrition* as well as numerous scientific articles, and also contributed chapters to the book *Rethink Food*. Dr. Stoll can be heard on his daily radio program, *Health Minutes,* in the Lehigh Valley, on Channel 60 TV's "health minutes," and in lectures nationally and internationally. He has also appeared on *The Dr. Oz Show, The Marilu Henner Show,* Trinity Broadcasting Network, and Daystar Television. Dr. Stoll and his wife, Kristen, live in Pennsylvania with their four sons and two daughters, where they, too, are actively involved in their church and community organizations.

$\mathcal{I}$ndex

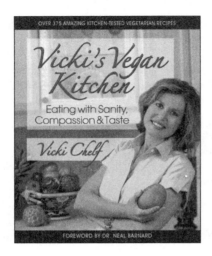

VICKI'S VEGAN KITCHEN
Eating with Sanity, Compassion & Taste
Vicki Chelf

Vegan dishes are healthy and delicious, yet many people are daunted by the idea of preparing meals that contain no animal products. For them, and for everyone who loves great food, vegetarian chef Vicki Chelf presents a comprehensive cookbook designed to take the mystery out of meatless meals. The book begins with an overview of the vegan diet and chapters on kitchen staples, cooking methods, and food preparation. Over 375 of Vicki's favorite recipes follow—and each one is easy to make and utterly delectable.

$17.95 US • 320 pages • 7.5 x 9-inch quality paperback • ISBN 978-0-7570-0251-9

ENEMY OF THE STEAK
Vegetarian Recipes to Win Friends and Influence Meat-Eaters
Nikki and David Goldbeck

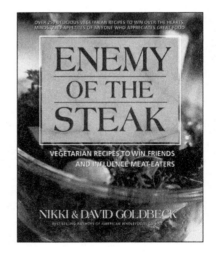

Enemy of the Steak is a wonderfully tempting vegetarian cookbook that offers a wealth of kitchen-tested recipes which nourish the body, please the palate, and satisfy even the heartiest of appetites. After presenting basics on vegetarian cooking, the book offers over 250 recipes for breakfast fare; appetizers and hors d'oeuvres; soups; salads; entrées; side dishes; sauces, toppings, and marinades; and desserts. A perfect marriage of nutrition and the art of cooking, *Enemy of the Steak* is for everyone who loves a good healthy meal.

$16.95 US • 248 pages • 7.5 x 9-inch quality paperback • ISBN 978-0-7570-0273-1

THE CHANGE COOKBOOK

Using the Power of Food to Transform Your Body, Your Health, and Your Life

Milan Ross and Scott Stoll, MD

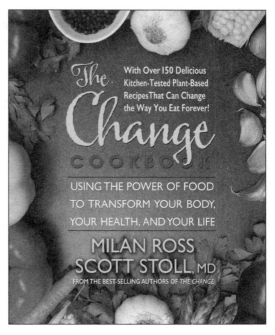

From the best-selling authors of *The Change* comes a new cookbook based on Dr. Stoll's Immersion program for weight loss and better health. Imagine dishes that can reduce your cholesterol, lower your blood pressure, boost your immune system, and decrease your odds of getting cancer, type 2 diabetes, heart disease, strokes, or a host of other all-too-common health problems. Here, in this new book, are over 150 recipes that can truly change your life for the better.

The book is divided into two parts. Part One begins with the journey taken by each author to develop such a cookbook. This section shares the plant-based food principles that have propelled their book *The Change* to become a bestseller. This is followed by an overview of a plant-based diet, including its nutritional benefits and impact on weight control. Subsequent chapters provide important information on kitchen staples, cooking methods, food preparation techniques, and helpful guidelines on shopping for the best-quality foods and ingredients.

In Part Two, the authors share over 150 kitchen-tested recipes for delectable dishes. Included are satisfying breakfast choices, luscious dips and spreads, sensational soups and salads, satisfying bean dishes, hearty pilafs and other grain creations, and veggie favorites, topped off with a collection of fantastic desserts. Each recipe provides easy-to-follow directions that ensure success.

December 2016 • $17.95 US • 256 pages • 7.5 x 9-inch quality paperback • ISBN 978-0-7570-0438-4

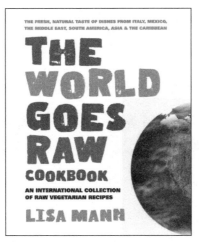

THE WORLD GOES RAW COOKBOOK
An International Collection of Raw Vegetarian Recipes

Although raw food can be delicious and improve your well-being, raw cuisine cookbooks have always offered little variety—until now. In *The World Goes Raw Cookbook,* chef Lisa Mann provides a fresh approach to (un)cooking. Lisa first guides you in stocking your kitchen and then presents six chapters of international dishes, including Italian, Mexican, Middle Eastern, Asian, Caribbean, and South American cuisine. Let *The World Goes Raw* add variety to your life while helping you feel healthier and more energized than ever before.

$16.95 US • 176 pages • 7.5 x 9-inch quality paperback • ISBN 978-0-7570-0320-2

EAT SMART, EAT RAW
Creative Vegetarian Recipes for a Healthier Life
Kate Wood

As the popularity of raw vegetarian cuisine soars, so does the evidence that uncooked food is amazingly good for you. Now there is another reason to go raw—taste! In *Eat Smart, Eat Raw,* Kate Wood presents 150 recipes for truly exceptional dishes, including hearty breakfasts, savory soups, satisfying entrées, and luscious desserts. Whether you

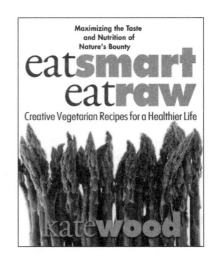

are an ardent vegetarian or just someone in search of a great meal, this book may forever change the way you look at an oven.

$15.95 US • 184 pages • 7.5 x 9-inch quality paperback • ISBN 978-0-7570-0261-8

GOING WILD IN THE KITCHEN
The Fresh & Sassy Tastes of Vegetarian Cooking
Leslie Cerier

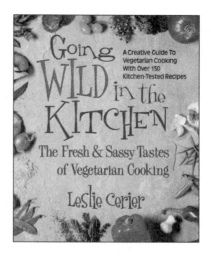

Venture beyond the usual beans, grains, and vegetables to include an exciting variety of organic vegetarian fare in your meals. *Going Wild in the Kitchen* shows you how. Author Leslie Cerier offers over 150 kitchen-tested recipes for taste-tempting dishes that contain such unique ingredients as edible flowers; wild mushrooms, berries, and herbs; and exotic ancient grains like teff, quinoa, and Chinese "forbidden" black rice. Leslie also encourages your creative instincts by prompting you to "go wild" and add new ingredients to existing recipes.

$16.95 US • 240 pages • 7.5 x 9-inch quality paperback • ISBN 978-0-7570-0091-1

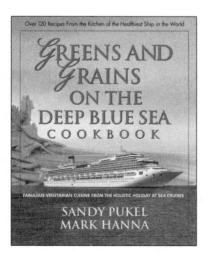

GREENS AND GRAINS ON THE DEEP BLUE SEA COOKBOOK
Fabulous Vegetarian Cuisine from the Holistic Holiday at Sea Cruises
Sandy Pukel and Mark Hanna

Come aboard one of America's premier health cruises. Can't get away? You can still enjoy its gourmet cuisine, because natural foods expert Sandy Pukel and master chef Mark Hanna have created *Greens and Grains on the Deep Blue Sea Cookbook*—a titanic collection of the most popular vegetarian dishes served aboard the Holistic Holiday at Sea cruises. Each of the book's more than 120 easy-to-follow recipes—from appetizers and entrées to side dishes and desserts—is designed to provide not only great taste, but also maximum nutrition.

$16.95 US • 160 pages • 7.5 x 9-inch quality paperback • ISBN 978-0-7570-0287-8

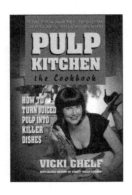

PULP KITCHEN:
THE COOKBOOK
How to Turn Juiced Pulp into Inspired Dishes
Vicki Chelf

In *Pulp Kitchen,* best-selling cookbook author Vicki Chelf shares the many uses for an often-overlooked ingredient—the high-fiber pulp that's a byproduct of juicing. Included are helpful preparation and storage guidelines plus dozens of kitchen-tested recipes that highlight pulp's versatility.

$14.95 US • 144 pages • 6 x 9-inch quality paperback • ISBN 978-0-7570-0396-7

JUICE ALIVE, SECOND EDITION
The Ultimate Guide to Juicing Remedies
Steven Bailey, ND, and Larry Trivieri, Jr.

In this easy-to-use guide, two health experts tell you everything you need to know to maximize the benefits of juicing. A chart matches up common ailments with the most appropriate juices, and 100 recipes make good nutrition completely delicious.

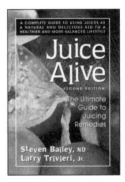

$14.95 US • 288 pages • 6 x 9-inch quality paperback • ISBN 978-0-7570-0266-3

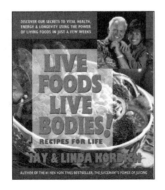

LIVE FOODS LIVE BODIES!
Jay and Linda Kordich

In *Live Foods Live Bodies!,* Jay and Linda Kordich reveal their secrets to healthful living, including juice therapy and a living foods diet. Lavishly illustrated, this powerful book features over 100 kitchen-tested recipes for delectable juices, salad dressings, soups, and more.

$18.95 US • 240 pages • 7.5 x 9-inch quality paperback • ISBN 978-0-7570-0385-1

THE ULTIMATE ALLERGY-FREE COOKBOOK

Over 150 Easy-to-Make Recipes That Contain No Milk, Eggs, Wheat, Peanuts, Tree Nuts, Soy, Fish, or Shellfish

Judi and Shari Zucker

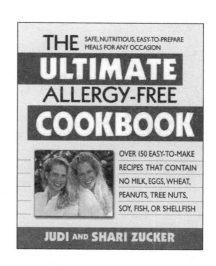

The Ultimate Allergy-Free Cookbook is an exciting collection of over 150 delectable dishes that contain absolutely no eggs, cow's milk, soy, wheat, peanuts, tree nuts, fish, or shellfish—the eight foods most likely to cause allergic reactions. It offers valuable information on the dangers of cross-contamination of allergens in packaged foods, and helps you understand food labels. You'll even learn how to stock a safe allergen-free kitchen.

$15.95 US • 192 pages • 7.5 x 9-inch quality paperback • ISBN 978-0-7570-0397-4

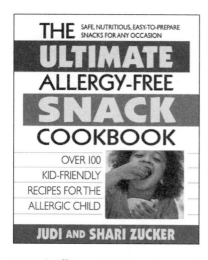

THE ULTIMATE ALLERGY-FREE SNACK COOKBOOK

Over 100 Kid-Friendly Recipes for the Allergic Child

Judi and Shari Zucker

Nearly all commercially made treats contain dairy, eggs, wheat (gluten), soy, peanuts, or tree nuts—the six ingredients that cause over 80 percent of all food allergies. To help parents gain some control, Judi and Shari Zucker have written *The Ultimate Allergy-Free Snack Cookbook,* a collection of over 100 nutritious and delicious allergen-free treats. It offers a complete recipe section of both sweet and savory kid-favorite choices, including chips, cookies, pizza, burgers, smoothies, and more. This really is the ultimate snack cookbook!

$15.95 US • 144 pages • 7.5 x 9-inch quality paperback • ISBN 978-0-7570-0346-2

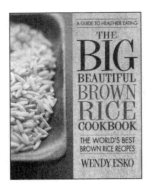

THE BIG BEAUTIFUL BROWN RICE COOKBOOK

The World's Best Brown Rice Recipes

Wendy Esko

When restaurants offer brown rice, the dish often appears bland and boring. But this grain can be as delectable as it is healthful. *The Big Beautiful Brown Rice Cookbook* features over 140 vegetarian/vegan recipes spotlighting this nutritional powerhouse.

$16.95 US • 192 pages • 7.5 x 9-inch quality paperback • ISBN 978-0-7570-0364-6

COOKING WITH SEITAN

The Complete Vegetarian "Wheat-Meat" Cookbook

Barbara Jacobs and Leonard Jacobs

Cooking with Seitan provides a wonderful introduction to this meat substitute and offers over 250 kitchen-tested recipes, featuring traditional and international favorites as well as new dishes, from salads to soups, stews, and even desserts.

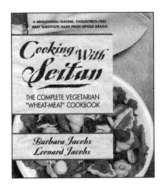

$17.95 US • 208 pages • 7.5 x 9-inch quality paperback • ISBN 978-0-7570-0304-2

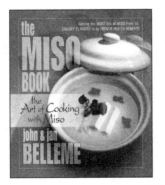

THE MISO BOOK

The Art of Cooking with Miso

John Belleme and Jan Belleme

For centuries, soybeans and grains have been transformed into miso, which is both a flavoring and a medicinal. *The Miso Book* begins with basic information and then presents over 140 recipes in which miso is used in dips, soups, and more.

$15.95 US • 192 pages • 7.5 x 9-inch quality paperback • ISBN 978-0-7570-0028-7

For more information about our books, visit our website at www.squareonepublishers.com